# Eat Fat Get Thin

## *For Rapid Weight Loss*

©*Samuel Cove*

# Forward

First, I would like to thank you for purchasing "Eat Fat Get Thin: For Rapid Weight Loss" and congratulate you for taking the leap to enhance your wellbeing and overall health.

In this book you will find scientifically proven strategies to help you lose weight in an efficient and sustainable way. Eating all natural, organic and nutrient dense foods that have high quality calories is the key to finding balance in your life and shedding the extra pounds once and for all.

Time and time again, scientific studies show that people on High Fat Low Carb Diets lose weight faster than people on Low-Fat diets… even when the low-fat dieters are actively restricting calories.

## Why?

Because eating FAT does not Make you FAT! Eating CARBS does!

By eating a diet high in healthy saturated fats you are sustained throughout the day. You don't get the sugar spikes and then sugar crashes.

You don't need the cake and coffee to stimulate you in the afternoon slump.

On this diet you'll be getting plenty of Good Fats from cold pressed oils, nuts and seeds, grass fed meat and eliminating all unnatural and processed foods.

This book will use a step-wise approach to take you through the high fat low carb diet and further beyond into the practical application of making healthy and super tasty recipes.

In this step-by step approach through the high fat low carb journey you will learn everything you need to know about this diet and beyond into the practical application of making delicious recipes. Expounding on a practical and sustainable ways to nourish our bodies, the high fat diet aims to maintain lifelong vibrancy, physical robustness and overall health.

As you embark on this journey towards health and vitality feel free to take notes as you go along as this is the diet that will change your life from now henceforth!

# Table of Contents

13

# The Truth About Fat

Of all the "nutritional myths" that have been spread by the mainstream media and FDA over the past few decades, one of the most harmful has been the idea that dietary fat, and specifically saturated fat, is responsible for weight gain and increased cardiovascular risk.
This fallacious idea has caused countless unknowing dieters to choose a "low-fat" diet with higher carbohydrate intake and has been the sole causal reason for insulin resistance and type 2 diabetes. In 1977, the all too familiar erroneous "Food Pyramid" release by the USDA was imposed on Americans and with it came an increase in carbohydrates and a decrease in consumption of saturated fat and cholesterol.
The guidelines for this "Food Pyramid" were based on studies that suggested that diets high in saturated fats increased the risk of coronary artery disease. This hypothesis has been debunked dozens of times through scientific review over the last 3 decades, yet this "Food Pyramid still remains in the present academic literature and is taught all over the States. Almost at the exact same time the obesity epidemic started in America began. This is more than just a mere coincidence.

## If Fat Doesn't Make People Fat, What Does?

Here's how the story plays out in your biology.
Sugar, in the form of carbohydrate or any other, spikes your fat-storing hormone **insulin**.
When you eat sugar, refined carbs or *anything* that raises your blood sugar, it causes a spike in your fat storage hormone– insulin. Then, a vicious cycle that includes hunger, cravings and overeating ensues.
Insulin drives all available fuel in your bloodstream into your fat cells, especially those around your tummy area AKA visceral fat, organ fat or most commonly, belly fat. This in turn stimulates your brain to make you eat more.
Another point of flaw is when to restrict calories and exercise more. Why does this strategy usually fail? Because your body becomes alarmed, fearing you're starving, and will tenaciously hang onto the fat reserves you already have due to the self-imposed famine.

## What is the High Fat Diet?

This is an eating plan that is built on a 30 day plan aimed at jumpstarting healthy lifestyle changes for the long run. It first starts by cleansing your body of all toxins that are weighing it down in readiness for the immense benefits of a nutrient-dense, organic and whole foods diet.

This is followed by delicious recipes that are built on protein and supplemented by high fat foods, super foods and spices bursting with flavor, fat-burning and health promoting results.

High fat low carb foods will help shred extra fat, they will boost your metabolism – rate at which your body burns calories and they will help you stay full after eating them – meaning you're going to eat less food. With the High fat low carb Diet we can finally say that we have solved the mystery of weight loss!

The High Fat Low Carb Diet is a simple approach to eating whole, unprocessed foods with a focus on nutrient rich vegetables, high-quality, unprocessed meats and heart healthy fats.

Most people on a low-fat diet end up taking in more carbs, especially processed ones, and in turn are hungry all the time. By filling up on whole, low carb foods and ditching the processed grains, sugars, and carbs, you will satiate your appetite while dropping the extra pounds. This diet will not only change the way you feel about food, it will also change your habits and your cravings. You will experience increased energy levels, improved mental focus and clarity, as well as better sleep. Sound too good to be true? Give it a try and see for yourself!

Whether you've never heard of the High Fat Low Carb Diet or you're a veteran who needs some inspiration when it comes to recipes, this book is here to help you to expand your horizons.

## Speed Up Your Metabolism with a High Fat Diet

In countless human experiments, those who ate high-fat, low carb diets had a much faster metabolism. In contrast, low-fat high-carb diets spike insulin, subsequently slowing their metabolism and storing dreaded belly fat. The higher-fat diet group had a faster metabolism, even when eating the exact same amount of calories. The faster your metabolic rate the more ability your body has to utilise the fat, adipose tissue and excess weight that you currently have. Keep this in mind as we go into the next chapters.

## Why Should I Avoid Carbs?

Refined grains and sugars are the biggest sources of carbs and a major cause of inflammation in the American diet, so these are the most important exclusions from the low carb high fat diet plan. High consumption of refined grains (white flour) and sugar is linked with higher risk for myriad diseases, everything from heart disease, stroke, Alzheimer's, and diabetes. Legumes are also high in starch, and they have certain types of fibre that are problematic for some people, so they too are excluded for this portion of the program. Dairy is another common source of dietary sensitivities, in addition to the fact that most milk products in the US today come from grain-fed cows, some of which are treated with hormones. Alcohol is also highly inflammatory, and linked with many serous health conditions.

By following this program for a month, you'll give yourself a chance to see how potentially problematic food groups like dairy, grains, and legumes are affecting your health. For some, eating moderate amounts of dairy and whole grains is no problem. Others can't, and experience symptoms like bloating, abdominal pain, and fatigue without knowing why. The only way to find out is to try at least a month without these foods and see how you feel. We suggest you experiment with the recipes in this book, but if your body does not agree with the dairy it is advised to omit these recipes from your diet.

Foods like refined grains and sugar are problematic for *everyone*, because they increase risk factors for chronic illnesses like heart disease, obesity, and diabetes. By cutting these out, you'll likely lose weight and reduce some of the related risk factors. Finally, by eating a lower-carb, medium protein, high fat diet, you'll also increase your body's capacity to burn fat as an energy source. Some research has shown that eating a diet lower in carbohydrates and higher in fat than the average American diet aids in weight loss and helps increase the body's ability to utilize fat stores as energy.

Another benefit is that the fat keeps you satiated for a much longer period of time. Say goodbye to those afternoon energy slumps and ravenous belly grumbles-healthy fat keeps you full for much longer! There are three other important parts of this program: drink plenty of water (your body needs to be fully hydrated in order to efficiently burn fat), get physical activity (at least 30 minutes to 1 hour every day. By eliminating grains and sugar, you will automatically eliminate most of the unhealthy foods in your diet, and very likely lose weight. But, sustainable weight loss takes weeks, not days. Your weight can fluctuate as much as 5 pounds in one day, and trying to track your progress with a scale on a daily basis will lead to added stress and take your focus away from the larger goal of better overall health.

Focus on maintaining the low carb high fat lifestyle and considerable weight loss will follow.

# The High Fat Goal

The goal is not to eat this diet for 30 days and then return to an average American diet full of processed food and soda. The idea is to build new habits that you can sustain for the rest of your life. A great opportunity for this is **finding new snack foods**. Americans tend to snack on a lot of sugary snacks full of refined grains and unhealthy fats. Cookies, candy bars, energy drinks, sodas…all of these provide a quick burst of energy – often leaving with a sugar crash half an hour later – but put you on the fast track to worse health in the future.

Try to find new snack combinations that are tasty, easy to prepare, and convenient to eat on the go. Decadent Fat Bombs, Hard boiled eggs, organic beef jerky, a handful or nuts and dried fruit, an apple with almond butter, raw vegetables dipped in homemade dressing, olives…there are dozens of options to keep you fuelled and on track. Check out the chapter on low carb snacks and make them in advanced so you have a batch for the entire week.

The low carb high fat diet emphasizes protein, but it's important to **choose your proteins thoughtfully**. The low carb high fat diet that is outlined in this book promotes a moderate amount of protein.

The reason for this is that excess protein consumed in the diet can get converted to carbohydrate through a complex process known as gluconeogenesis, thereby preventing weight loss

As much as you can, focus on chicken, turkey, fish, and eggs to supply lean protein in your diet. When you buy beef or lamb, it's very important to get organic, 100% grass-fed meat. Research has shown that the type of fat differs in grass-fed and grain-fed meats as the grain that is fed is usually genetically modified and filled with hormones which can cause various health conditions

Decide what you're going to cook a few days in advance, so you can prep ingredients ahead of time and have meals and snacks ready *before* you get super hungry. Slow-cooker stews can be started in the morning and will be ready when you get home from work. Many dishes can be made the day before and reheated. Most can even be frozen. And things like salads are often quick to throw together. Knowing what you have on hand and what you'll make with it will help you stick to your low carb high fat diet.

As part of planning ahead, **take any high carbohydrate foods out of your house**, or at the very least, put them out of sight and each reach. This month will be challenging at times, and you can make it easier on yourself by making it harder to break the rules. You're more likely to eat cookies that you left sitting on your counter than to get dressed, drive to the store, and buy cookies. Our willpower is limited, so remove temptation ahead of time when you can.

It may be challenging, but the low carb high fat diet is a great chance to try **new foods and recipes**. Look for recipes from cuisines that don't typically use a lot of grains or legumes, like Thai or Chinese stir-fries and South Asian curries. Take a familiar low carb high fat diet friendly dish, like beef stew or scrambled eggs, and look for ways to give it a fresh twist with new spices, a different mixture of vegetables, or another culture's take on it.

Finally, **surround yourself with support**. Team up with a friend, spouse, or co-worker who wants to try the low carb high fat diet. You'll be less likely to stop if you're doing it with someone else. Look up the dozens of low carb high fat diet blogs and forums online and join the virtual community. Plan rewards for yourself through the month that don't involve food: a movie, sleeping in, dates with friends, a trip to your favourite store – whatever it is that gives you motivation. Good luck on this valuable step to a healthier you.

## Detoxifying the Natural Way

Feeling out of sync or sluggish? Are you in constant battle with fatigue, skin breakouts, aches, unexplainable pains and digestive problems and not forgetting, a constant struggle with weight loss? Well, your body is placing a distress call and it's about time for a great detox.

This is the first thing you should do before embarking on the low carb high fat diet. For faster health and weight loss results, you should first cleanse your system.

As with all the principles of the low carb high fat diet, we are going to do the detox au natural. By removing and eliminating all toxins from your body and feeding on a fresh, natural and wholesome diet, you will not only protect your body from disease but you will also renew your ability to attain optimum health and set yourself up for successful and sustainable weight loss.

## Cleansing and detoxifying naturally

Basically, cleansing and detoxifications means cleaning your blood. This is achieved by removing impurities and free radicals from the blood in your liver, where toxins are usually processed for elimination. Your body also eliminates toxins through your intestines, kidneys, lymph's, lungs and skin.

However, when your body is compromised, impurities are not filtered in the right way and every cell in your body is adversely affected.

A healthy detox program helps your body's natural cleansing process by:

- Stimulating your liver to eliminate toxins from your body
- Resting your organs through periodic fasting
- Improving your blood circulation
- Promoting elimination of toxins through your kidneys, intestines and skin; and
- Rejuvenating your body with healthy high fat foods

The reason natural detoxification works is because it addresses the specific needs of individual cells which are the smallest units of human life.

## How do you know that your body needs detoxification?

Today, with more toxins in our environment than ever before, it's essential to detox in order to keep our bodies functioning smoothly. We recommend that you detox your body at least once a year. You know that you need to detox if you experience symptoms such as:

- Allergies
- Unexplained fatigue
- Regular bloating
- Menstrual irregularities
- Sluggish elimination
- Mental confusion such as memory lapses
- Irritated skin
- Puffy eyes

24

# How to detox

The first step is to lighten your toxic load by eliminating all processed foods (refined and artificial and sugars, refined and bleached flours, hydrogenated and trans fats, gluten, chemicals in food and genetically modified foods), cigarettes, alcohol and coffee, all of which are received as toxins by your body and are an obstacle to the normal functioning of your body.

You should also minimize or better yet, eliminate the use of chemical-based detergents, household products, deodorant, and skin care products; and substitute them with organic and all natural alternatives. Stress is another deterrent to good health as it triggers the release of stress hormones in your system. In large amounts these stress hormones override your detoxification enzymes in your liver. Meditation and yoga are some of the methods to help you deal with stress the right way.

## The best ways to help your body detoxify

1. Drink at least eight glasses of water a day.
2. Eat plenty of negative calorie foods that are high fibre and that are organically grown. Radish, beets and edible seaweed are detoxifying super foods.
3. Take vitamin C rich foods. Vitamin C helps your body produce glutathione, a liver compound that eliminates toxins.
4. Cleanse and protect your liver by taking herbs such as milk thistle, dandelion root and burdock
5. Practice swimmers breathing (deep breathing) to allow oxygen to circulate more effectively and completely through your system.
6. Go to a sauna to allow your body to eliminate toxins through perspiration
7. Occasionally practice hydrotherapy by taking an extremely hot shower (as hot as you can handle) for five minutes; allowing the water to run down your body, especially your back. Follow this with very cold water for 30 seconds. Repeat this 3 times then take a nap for 30 minutes.
8. Dry brush your skin to drive toxins through your pores – look for special brushes in natural products department stores.

9. Exercising is a great way to detoxify. Fast jump roping and yoga are very effective. 30 minutes every day is enough time for an effective workout.

## All day fat flushing tea

1. Combine 8 cups of brewed green tea (unsweetened) with slices of lime, lemon and orange in a large pitcher.
2. Serve over ice or take it hot. You can refrigerate for up to 3 days.
3. Take 1 pitcher of this fat flushing tea a day for 5 days.

Give natural cleansing and detoxification an honest try and you are going to love how the low carb high fat diet is going to work for you in your weight loss journey and also in helping you transition to healthier long term eating habits.

We are now going to jump to the fun part of the book – FOOD!

We are doing all the work for you by sharing with you a 1 FULL Month meal plan that features some of the healthiest and tastiest recipes you've ever tasted. But first, get your apron ready and let's get cooking!

# One Full Month Meal Plan

You've heard it said; 'failure to plan is planning to fail.' Whether you are only cooking for one or for your entire family, taking the time to sit and plan for what you are going to eat for the coming week will not just save you time, money and effort; it will also enhance your healthy eating habits.

## Four reasons why you should have a meal plan:

- **You will culture healthy eating habits**

The main premise of The High Fat Diet is to eat food that is going to help your body burn fat and also protect you from disease by keeping your immune system strong. When you have a carefully set out meal plan, you won't need to resort to ordering takeout as you will have healthy food waiting for you at home.

Habit is second to nature and as you get used to planning healthy meals, you will soon forget about the processed and inflammatory foods that used to slow you down.

- **You become an informed shopper**

The specific ingredients listed in the recipes you are going to make will teach you the healthiest ingredients that you need to buy. Forget about overly processed food that has got no nutritional value, you focus will now shift to fresh, natural, nutrient dense foods.

- **You will save time and money**

When you know exactly what you are going to cook, you will shop for ingredients more efficiently and thus save more money. You won't also have to waste time brainstorming on what to cook as it's already planned.

- **You will eat a variety of food**

Planning your meals will allow you to eat something new almost every day, if not every day, instead of eating one thing all week. If you have a family, they are sure to dig this method and it will give them something to look forward to every day.

27

| Meal Plan – Week One | | | |
|---|---|---|---|
| | **Monday** | **Tuesday** | **Wednesday** |
| **Breakfast** | Anaheim pepper Gruyere Waffles | Anchovy, Spinach and Asparagus Omelet | Mahón Kale Sausage Omelet Pie |
| **Lunch** | Baked Creamy Cauliflower-Broccoli Chicken | Baked Manchego Chicken Wings | Baked Pork Chops in Sweet-Sour Marinade |
| **Dinner** | Chicken & Endive Casserole | Creamy Smoked Turkey Salad with Almonds | Herb Baked Salmon Fillets |
| **Thursday** | **Friday** | **Saturday** | **Sunday** |
| Monterey Bacon-Scallions Omelet | Smoked Turkey Bacon and Avocado Muffins | Sour Cream Cheese Pancakes | Spicy Cauliflower with Sujuk Sausages |
| Bolognese Squash Spaghetti | Cheesy Zoodles with Fresh Basil | Spicy Spinach Casserole | Slow Cooker Roast and Chicken Stew |
| Beef Cabbage Parsley Soup | Boneless Lamb Stew | Butternut Squash Soup | Duck Breast with Balsamic Vinegar |

| Meal Plan – Week Two | | | |
|---|---|---|---|
| | Monday | Tuesday | Wednesday |
| **Breakfast** | Vesuvius Scrambled Eggs with Provolone | Cheesy Bacon and Chive Omelet | Breakfast Quiche |
| **Lunch** | Mediterranean Pecorino Romano Breaded Cutlets | Oriental Garlicky Chicken Thighs | Pordenone Cauliflower Lasagna |
| **Dinner** | Hot Mexican Meatballs | Lamb Cutlets with Garlic Sauce | Slow Cooker Buffalo Chicken |
| Thursday | Friday | Saturday | Sunday |
| Bacon Avocado Breakfast Muffins | Chicharrones con Huevos (Pork Rind & Eggs) | Red Pepper, Mozzarella and Bacon Frittata | Vanilla Chia Oatmeal |
| Roasted Chicken & Prosciutto with Brussels sprouts | Roquefort Spinach, Zoodles and Bacon Salad | Sour Avocado and Chicken Moussaka | Spicy Italian Sausage and Spinach Casserole |
| Spinach Soup with Almonds and Parmesan | Slow Cooker Thai Fish Curry | Seafood Stew | Chicken Stir-Fry |

| Meal Plan – Week Three | | | |
|---|---|---|---|
| | Monday | Tuesday | Wednesday |
| **Breakfast** | Breakfast Taco | Raspberry & Cacao Breakfast Pudding | Caprese Stack |
| **Lunch** | Squash Spaghetti Lasagna Dish | Tuna Avocado Bites | Crispy Baked Tofu and Bok Choy Salad |
| **Dinner** | Pan Fried Hake | Bell Peppers Stuffed Korean Beef | Creamy Tarragon Chicken |
| **Thursday** | **Friday** | **Saturday** | **Sunday** |
| Easy Pancakes | Veggie Scramble | Egg Pesto Scramble | Lemon Cheesecake Breakfast Mousse |
| Homemade Meatballs | BBQ Chicken Soup | Bacon Chicken Patties | Savory Mince |
| Beanless Chili con Carne | Seared Ribeye Steak | Italian Fish Stew | Chicken and Mushroom Stew |

| Meal Plan – Week Four | | | |
|---|---|---|---|
| | **Monday** | **Tuesday** | **Wednesday** |
| **Breakfast** | Mozzarella, Red Pepper & Bacon Frittata | Rosemary, Sausage & Cheese Pies | Bacon, Scallions & Monterey Omelet |
| **Lunch** | Beef Sausage, Bacon & Broccoli Casserole | Hearty Portobello Burgers | Chicken and Broccoli filled Zucchini |
| **Dinner** | Beef Shin Stew | Bacon, Beef Sausage and Broccoli Casserole | Creamy Haddock |
| **Thursday** | **Friday** | **Saturday** | **Sunday** |
| Choco Moko Chia Porridge | Hemp Muffins with Walnuts | Boiled Eggs with Mascarpone and Bacon | Pork and Sage Breakfast Burgers |
| Salmon Salad in Avocado Cups | Beef Shred Salad | Spicy Chicken Thighs | Slow Cooker Chicken Stew |
| Baked Herb Salmon Fillets | Lamb Cutlets with Garlic Sauce | Tender Pork & Bacon Cassoulet | Ratatouille |

# Breakfast Recipe

# Mahón Kale Sausage Omelet Pie

**Ingredients**

10 eggs

1 1/2 cup Mahón cheese (or Cheddar)

3 chicken sausages

3 cups raw chopped Kale leaves

2 1/2 cup mushrooms, chopped

1 Tbsp. garlic powder

2 tsp. hot sauce

1/2 tsp. black pepper and celery seed

salt and pepper to taste

**Directions**

1. Preheat oven to 400F.
2. Chop up your sausage and mushroom thin and place them in a cast iron skillet. Cook on a medium-high heat for 2-3 minutes.
3. While the sausages are cooking, chop your spinach up. Add in a skillet the mushrooms and spinach.
4. In a meanwhile, in a bowl mix eggs with black pepper and celery seed, hot sauce, and spices. Scramble them well.
5. Mix your sausages, spinach, and mushrooms so that the spinach can wilt fully. Add salt and pepper to taste.
6. Finally, add the cheese to the top.
7. Pour your eggs over the mixture and mix everything well.
8. Stir the mixture for a few seconds, and then put your cast iron skillet in the oven. Bake for 10-12 minutes, and then broil the top for 3-4 minutes.
9. Let cool for a while, cut into 8 slices and serve hot.

Servings: 8

Cooking Times: 25 minutes

**Nutrition Facts (per serving)**

Calories 266

Fat 17,76g

Carbs 7,67g

Fiber 0,92g

Protein 19,37g

# Monterey Bacon-Scallions Omelet

### Ingredients
2 eggs
2 slices cooked bacon
1/4 cup scallions, chopped
1/4 cup Monterey jack cheese
Salt and pepper to taste
1 tsp. lard

### Directions
1. In a frying pan heat lard in on medium-low heat. Add the eggs, scallions and salt and pepper to taste.
2. Cook for 1-2 minutes; add the bacon and sauté 30 - 45 seconds longer. Turn the heat off on the stove.
3. On top of the bacon place a cheese. Then, take two edges of the omelet and fold them onto the cheese. Hold the edges there for a moment as the cheese has to partially melt. Make the same with the other egg and let cook in a warm pan for a while.
4. Serve hot.

Servings: 2

Cooking Times
Total Time: 15 minutes

### Nutrition Facts (per serving)
Calories 321
Fat 28,31g
Carbs 1,62g
Fiber 0,33g
Protein 14,37g

# Smoked Turkey Bacon and Avocado Muffins

**Ingredients**

5 eggs

6 slices smoked turkey bacon

1/2 cup almond flour

2 medium Avocados

1/2 cup Cheddar cheese

1 1/2 cup coconut milk

3 spring onions

1 tsp. minced garlic

2 tsp. dried parsley

1/4 tsp. red chili powder

1 1/2 Tbsp. lemon juice

1/4 cup flaxseed

1 1/2 Tbsp. Metamucil powder

1 tsp. baking powder

2 Tbsp. butter

Salt and pepper to taste

**Directions**

1.  Preheat oven to 350F.
2.  In a frying pan over medium-low heat, cook the bacon with the butter until crisp. Add the spring onions, cheese, and baking powder.
3.  In a bowl, mix together coconut milk, eggs, Metamucil powder, almond flour, flax, spices and lemon juice. Switch off the heat & let cool. Crumble the bacon & add all of the fat to the egg mixture.
4.  Clean and chop avocado and fold into the mixture.
5.  Measure out batter into a cupcake tray that's been sprayed or greased with nonstick spray and bake for 25-26 minutes.
6.  Once ready, let cool and serve hot or cold.

Servings: 16

Cooking Times: 40 minutes

**Nutrition Facts (per serving)**

Calories 184

Fat 16,4g

Carbs 5,51g

Fiber 2,7g

Protein 5,89g

# Sour Cream Cheese Pancakes

### Ingredients
2 eggs
1/4 cup cream cheese
1 Tbsp. coconut flour
1 tsp. ground ginger
1/2 cup liquid Stevia
Coconut oil
Sugar-free maple syrup

### Directions
1. In a deep bowl, beat together all of the ingredients until smooth.
2. Heat up a frying skillet with oil on medium-high. Ladle the batter and pour in hot oil.
3. Cook on one side and then flip. Top with a sugar-free maple syrup and serve.

Servings: 2

Cooking Times
Total Time: 15 minutes

### Nutrition Facts (per serving)
Calories 170
Fat 13,71g
Carbs 4,39g
Fiber 0,14g
Protein 6,9g

# Spicy Cauliflower with Sujuk Sausages

## Ingredients

4 cups frozen cauliflower

8 oz. sujuk sausages sliced (or red pastrami)

1 green pepper, chopped

1 tsp. Cajun seasoning

1/2 onion, chopped

2 Tbsp. minced garlic

2 Tbsp. olive oil

## Directions

1. In a frying pan, sauté onion with olive oil for 2-3 minutes.
2. Squeeze the liquid from chopped cauliflower and add it to the pan. Sauté the cauliflower with onion 5-10 minutes.
3. Add in Cajun seasoning and mix. Add in chopped sujuk sausages or pastrami and green peppers.
4. Toss and cook until about 5 minutes. Transfer to the plates. Serve.

Servings: 4

Cooking Times
Total Time: 20 minutes

## Nutrition Facts (per serving)

Calories 181,

Fat 10,21g

Carbs 9,52g

Fiber 2,77g

Protein 14g

# Strawberry Marjoram Smoothie

### Ingredients
1/4 cup fresh or frozen strawberries
2 fresh marjoram leaves
2 Tbsp. heavy cream
1 cup unsweetened coconut milk
1 Tbsp. sugar-free vanilla syrup
1/2 tsp. pure vanilla extract
ice cubes (optional)

### Directions
1. Place all ingredients in your blender and mix until become smooth.
2. If you wish you can add the ice cubes. Serve.

Servings: 1
Cooking Time: 5 minutes

### Nutrition Facts (per serving)
Calories 292, 35
Fat 29,75g
Carbs 6,78g
Protein 2,84g

# Vesuvius Scrambled Eggs with Provolone

### Ingredients
2 large eggs
3/4 cup Provolone cheese
1.76 oz. air-dried salami
1 tsp. fresh rosemary (chopped)
1 Tbsp. Olive oil
Salt and pepper to taste

### Directions
1. In a small pan with olive oil fry the chopped salami.
2. In the meantime, in a small bowl whisk the eggs, then add the salt, pepper and fresh rosemary.
3. Add in the provolone cheese and mix well with a fork.
4. Pour the egg mixture to the pan with salami and cook for about 5 minutes. Serve hot.

Servings: 2

Cooking Time: 10 minutes

### Nutrition Facts (per serving)
Calories 374
Fat 30,32g
Total Carbs 2,43g
Fiber 0,27g
Protein 22,45g

# Pizza Waffles

## Ingredients
Parmesan cheese (4 tablespoons)
Psyllium husk powder (1 tablespoon)
Baking powder (1 teaspoon)
Salt
Cheddar cheese (3 oz.)
Eggs (4, large)
Almond flour (3 tablespoons)
Butter (1 tablespoon, organic)
Italian seasoning (1 teaspoon)-you may use a teaspoon of your preferred spices
Tomato sauce (1/2 cup)

## Directions
1. Add all ingredients to a bowl except cheese and tomato sauce. Use mixer or immersion blender to combine until mixture is thick.
2. Heat waffle iron and use mixture to make two waffles.
3. Place waffles onto a lined baking sheet and top with tomato sauce and cheese (divide evenly). Broil for 3 minutes or until cheese melts.
4. Serve.

Servings: 2

## Nutrition Facts (per serving)
Calories 525
Net Carbs 5g
Fats 41.5g
Protein 29g
Fiber 5.5g

# Pancakes and Syrup

**Ingredients**

*For pancakes:*
Eggs (4, large)
Erythritol (2 tablespoons)
Baking soda (1/2 teaspoon)
Nut butter of your choice (3/4 cup)
Coconut milk (1/3 cup)
Ghee (2 tablespoons)
Cinnamon powder (1 teaspoon)

*For Syrup:*
Maple extract (2 tablespoons, sugar-free)
Sukrin Fiber Syrup (1/2 cup)

**Directions**
1. Add ingredients for syrup to a jar and use spoon to stir until combined thoroughly. Cover jar and put aside until needed.
2. Put eggs, erythritol, baking soda, nut butter, coconut milk and cinnamon powder in a food processor and pulse until blended.
3. Heat ghee in a non-stick skillet and add batter to pot, use about ¼ cup per pancake. Cook until pancake sets then flip and finish cooking; place on a plate.
4. Repeat with remaining batter and plate.
5. Top with syrup and serve.

Servings: 5

**Nutrition Facts (per serving)**
Calories 401
Net Carbs 3.6g
Fats 32.5g
Protein 12.8g
Fiber 5.3g

# Cheesy Bacon and Chive Omelet

### Ingredients
Bacon fat (1 teaspoon)
Cheddar cheese (1 oz.)
Salt
Bacon (2 slices, cooked)
Eggs (2, large)
Black pepper
Chives (2 stalks)

### Directions
1. Beat eggs together and add pepper and salt to taste. Chop chives and shred cheese.
2. Heat skillet and cook bacon fat until hot.
3. Add eggs to pot and top with chives. Cook until edges start to set then add bacon and cook for 30-60 seconds.
4. Add cheese and use spatula to fold in half. Press to seal and flip over.
5. Warm and serve immediately.

Servings: 1

### Nutrition Facts (per serving)
Calories 463
Net Carbs 1g
Fats 39g
Protein 24g
Fiber 0g

# Breakfast Quiche

## Ingredients
Coconut oil (3 tablespoons)
5 whole eggs
8 slices of bacon, cooked and chopped
100ml cream
Baby spinach, roughly chopped (2 cups)
Red pepper, chopped (1 cup)
Green pepper, chopped (1 cup)
Yellow onion, chopped (1 cup)
2 cloves of garlic, minced
Mushrooms, chopped (1 cup)
100g cheddar cheese, grated
Salt to taste

## Directions
1. Preheat oven at 375F
2. In a large bowl, mix all vegetables including the mushrooms together.
3. In another small bowl, whisk the 5 eggs with the cream
4. Carefully scoop the veggie mixture into a muffin pan coated with cooking spray, top with egg and cheese filling up to ¾ of the muffin tins. Sprinkle with chopped bacon on top.
5. Place in the oven to bake for 15 minutes or until the top of the quiche are firm.
6. Let it cook for a few minutes before serving.

Servings: 5

## Nutrition Facts (per serving)
Calories: 210
Net Carbs: 5g
Fat: 13g
Protein: 6g

43

# Bacon Avocado Breakfast Muffins

**Ingredients**
Bacon (5 slices)
Almond flour (1/2 cup)
Psyllium husk powder (1 ½ tablespoons)
Colby Jack cheese (4.5 oz.)
Garlic (1 teaspoon, diced)
Chives (1 teaspoon, dried)
Lemon juice (1 ½ tablespoons)
Eggs (5)
Butter (2 tablespoons, organic)
Flaxseed meal (1/4 cup)
Avocados (2, cubed)
Spring onions (3)
Cilantro (1 teaspoon, dried)
Red chili flakes (1/4 teaspoon)
Coconut milk (1 ½ cup, from box)
Salt & Black Pepper
Baking powder (1 teaspoon)

**Directions**
1. Add flour, spices, lemon juice, eggs, flaxseed meal and coconut milk to a bowl. Mix together until thoroughly combined.
2. Heat a skillet and cook bacon until crispy then add the butter and avocado.
3. Add mixture to batter in bowl and mix together.
4. Set oven to 350 F and grease cupcake molds.
5. Add batter to molds and bake for 26 minutes. Take from oven and cool before removing from mold. Serve. Store leftovers in fridge.

Servings: 16

**Nutrition Facts (per serving)**
Calories 163
Net Carbs 1.5g
Fats 14.1g
Protein 6.1g
Fiber 3.3g

# Chicharrones con Huevos (Pork Rind & Eggs)

**Ingredients**
Bacon (4 slices)
Pork Rinds (1.5 oz.)
Avocado (1, cubed)
Onion (1/4, chopped)
Salt
Eggs (5)
Tomato (1, chopped)
Jalapeno pepper (2, seeds removed and chopped)
Cilantro (1/4 cup, chopped)
Black pepper

**Directions**
1. Heat skillet and cook bacon until slightly crisp. Remove from pot and put aside on paper towels.
2. Add pork rinds to pot along with onion, tomatoes, pepper and cook for 3 minutes until onions are soft and clear.
3. Add cilantro, stir together gently and add eggs. Scramble eggs and then add avocado and fold.
4. Serve.

Servings: 3

**Nutrition Facts (per serving)**
Calories 508
Net Carbs 5g
Fats 43g
Protein 24.7g
Fiber 5.3g

# Red Pepper, Mozzarella and Bacon Frittata

**Ingredients**

Olive oil (1 tablespoon)
Parsley (2 tablespoons, chopped)
Mozzarella cheese (4 oz., cubed)
Bell pepper (1, red, chopped)
Heavy cream (1/4 cup)
Bacon (7 slices)
Bella mushrooms (4 caps, large)
Basil (1/2 cup, chopped)
Goat cheese (2 oz., grated)
Eggs (9)
Parmesan cheese (1/4 cup, grated)
Salt & Black pepper

**Directions**

1. Set oven to 350 °F.
2. Chop red pepper, bacon, basil and mushroom. Slice mozzarella into cubes and put aside.
3. Heat olive oil in a skillet until it slightly smokes then add bacon and cook for 5 minutes until browned.
4. Add red pepper and cook for 2 minutes until soft. While pepper cooks, add cream, parmesan cheese, eggs and black pepper to a bowl and whisk to combine.
5. Add mushrooms to pot, stir and cook for 5 minutes until soaked in fat. Add basil, cook for 1 minute then add mozzarella.
6. Put in egg mixture and use spoon to move ingredients around so that the egg gets on the bottom of pan.
7. Top with goat cheese and place in oven for 8 minutes then broil for 6 minutes.
8. Use knife to pry frittata edges from pan and place on a plate and slice. Serve.

Servings: 6

**Nutrition Facts (per serving)**

Calories 408
Net Carbs 2.4g
Fats 31.2g
Protein 19.2g

46

# Cheese and Sausage Pies

**Ingredients**
Cheddar cheese (3/4 cup, grated)
Coconut oil (1/4 cup)
Egg yolks (5)
Rosemary (1/2 teaspoon)
Baking soda (1/4 teaspoon)
Chicken sausage (1 ½)
Coconut flour (1/4 cup)
Coconut milk (2 tablespoons)
Lemon juice (2 teaspoons)
Cayenne pepper (1/4 teaspoon)
Kosher salt (1/8 teaspoon)

**Directions**
1. Set oven to 350 °F.
2. Chop sausage, heat skillet and cook sausage. While sausages cook combine all dry ingredients in a bowl. In another bowl combine lemon juice, oil and coconut milk. Add liquids to dry mixture and add ½ cup of cheese; fold to combine and put into 2 ramekins.
3. Add cooked sausages to batter and use spoon to push into mixture.
4. Bake for 25 minutes until golden on top. Top with leftover cheese and broil for 4 minutes.
5. Serve warm.

Servings: 2

**Nutrition Facts (per serving)**
Calories 711
Net Carbs 5.8g
Fats 65.3g
Protein 34.3g
Fiber 11.5g

# Vanilla Chia Oatmeal

### Ingredients
Chia seeds (1/4 cup)
Coconut flakes (1/3 cup, unsweetened)
Vanilla (1 teaspoon, sugar free)
Almond milk (1 cup, unsweetened)
Stevia extract (10 drops)
Coconut (1/4 cup, shredded, unsweetened)
Almonds (1/3 cup, flaked)
Heavy whipping cream (1/2 cup)
Erythritol (2 tablespoons)

### Directions
1. Place almond and coconut flakes in a pot and toast for 3 minutes until fragrant.
2. Place toasted ingredients into a bowl along with chia seeds, erythritol and shredded coconut; mix together to combine.
3. Top with milk and stir. You can use hot or cold milk based on your preference.
4. Add vanilla and stevia, stir and set aside for 5-10 minutes.
5. Serve. May be topped with fresh berries.

Servings: 2

### Nutrition Facts (per serving)
Calories 359
Net Carbs 5g
Fats 30.4g
Protein 9.4 g
Fiber 10.5g

# Breakfast Berry Shake

## Ingredients

Mixed berries (3/4 cup)
Almond milk (1 cup)
All-natural peanut butter (1 tablespoon)
Protein powder (1 tablespoon)
Cinnamon powder (1/4 teaspoons)
Ginger, minced (1/4 teaspoons)

## Directions

1. Place all the ingredients in a blender and mix until smooth.

Servings: 3

## Nutrition Facts (per serving)

Calories: 319
Net Carbs: 9g
Fat: 15g
Protein: 28g

# Breakfast Tacos

### Ingredients
Eggs (6)
Bacon (3 strips)
Cheddar cheese (1 oz., shredded)
Mozzarella cheese (1 cup, shredded)
Butter (2 tablespoons)
Avocado (1/2, cubed)
Salt
Black pepper

### Directions
1. Cook bacon until crisp, put aside until needed.
2. Heat a non-stick pan and place 1/3 cup mozzarella into pan and cook for 3 minutes until browned around the edges. Place a wooden spoon across a bowl or pot and use tongs to lift cheese 'taco from pot. Repeat with leftover cheese.
3. Melt butter in a skillet and scramble eggs; use pepper and salt to season.
4. Spoon eggs into hardened shells and top with avocado and bacon.
5. Top with cheddar and serve.

Servings: 2

### Nutrition Facts (per serving)
Calories 443
Net Carbs 3g
Fats 36.2g
Protein 25.7 g
Fiber 1.7g

# Raspberry & Cacao Breakfast Pudding

**Ingredients**

Cacao powder (1 tablespoon)
Raspberry (1/4 cups)
Chia seeds (3 tablespoon)
Almond milk (1 cup)
Agave or Xylitol (1 teaspoon)

**Directions**

1.  In a small bowl, combine the almond milk and cacao powder. Stir well.
2.  Add the chia seeds to the bowl and let it rest for 5 minutes.
3.  Using a fork, fluff the chia and cacao mixture and then place in the fridge to chill for at least 30 minutes.
4.  Serve with raspberries and a drizzle of agave on top

Servings: 1

**Nutrition Facts (per serving)**

Calories 230
Net Carbs 4g
Fats 20g
Protein 15 g

# Orange Cinnamon Scones

**Ingredients**

*For Scones:*
Heavy cream (1/3 cup)
Butter (1/4 cup, unsalted, cubed)
Coconut oil (2 tablespoons)
Golden Flaxseed (1 tablespoon)
Cinnamon (1 ½ teaspoons)
Xanthan (1/4 teaspoon)
Salt (1/4 teaspoon)
Coconut flour (8 tablespoons)
Erythitol (1/4 cup)
Eggs (2)
Maple syrup (2 tablespoons)-recipe above
Baking powder (1 ½ teaspoons)
Vanilla (1 teaspoon)
Stevia (1/4 teaspoon)
Orange zest (from 1 orange)

*For Icing:*
Stevia (20 drops)
Orange juice (1 tablespoon)
Coconut butter (1/4 cup)

**Directions**
1. Set oven to 400 F.
2. Place all dry ingredients in a bowl except xanthan and 1 tablespoon flour. Add butter and oil to dry mix and stir to combine.
3. Combine sweetener and eggs until thoroughly mixed and light in color. Put in maple syrup, remaining flour, xanthan gum, heavy cream and vanilla; mix until combined and thick.
4. Add wet mixture to dry, reserving 2 tablespoons of liquids, mix together and add cinnamon and use hands to form mixture into dough. Shape into a ball and press into a cake like shape. Slice into 8 pieces.
5. Place onto a lined baking sheet and use reserved liquid to brush the top of scones.

6. Bake for 15 minutes, remove from oven and cool.
7. Prepare icing and drizzle over scones before serving.

Servings: 8

**Nutrition Facts (per serving)**
Calories 232
Net Carbs 3.3g
Fats 20g
Protein 3.3 g
Fiber 4.3g

# Buttermilk Seed Rusks

**Ingredients**

½ cup butter, melted

1 cup buttermilk

4 eggs

1 cup almond flour

1 cup ground flax

2 cups desiccated coconut

1 cup mixed seeds

2 ½ tsp. baking powder

1 tsp. salt

½ cup Xylitol

**Directions**

1. Preheat oven at 350F
2. In a bowl, combine the yogurt, butter, and eggs.
3. Slowly add the dry ingredients and stir well to make a batter.
4. Carefully transfer the mixture into a baking tray and cook in the oven for 45 minutes.
5. Allow to cool down before slicing it into 30 rusk shapes.
6. Place on a wire rack upside down, and cook in the oven again for 90 minutes at 210F.

Servings: 30

**Nutrition Facts** (1 rusk)

Calories: 119

Net Carbs: 17g

Fat: 3g

Protein: 2g

# Caprese Stack

**Ingredients**
3 slices mozzarella cheese
2 large slices of tomato
4 fresh basil leaves
salt and pepper
1 tsp. olive oil

**Directions**
1. On a plate, stack the mozzarella cheese, tomato, and basil.
2. Season with salt and pepper and drizzle with olive oil

**Nutrition Facts** (per stack)
Calories: 186
Net Carbs: 5g
Fat: 10g
Protein: 6g

# Easy Pancakes

### Ingredients
1 tbsp. melted butter
2 eggs
5 tbsp. full-fat milk
1 tbsp. xylitol
½ tsp. salt
2 tbsp. coconut flour
1 tbsp. almond flour
½ tsp. baking powder

### Directions
1. In a bowl, whisk the eggs with the milk, salt, xylitol, and melted butter (room temp.)
2. Add the coconut and almond flour to the mixture, along with the baking powder. Mix well.
3. Heat a non-stick pan over medium fire and scoop 3 tbsp. of the batter to make pancakes.
4. Flip the pancake when bubbles start to form and cook until golden brown.
5. Serve with ½ cup of berries on the side.

Servings: 2

**Nutrition Facts** (1 pc.)
Calories: 194
Net Carbs: 30g
Fat: 13g
Protein: 31g

# Mug Bread

**Ingredients**

1 tbsp. coconut flour
3 tbsp. almond flour
1 tsp. baking powder
1 whole egg
1 tsp. melted butter
3 tbsp. water
a pinch of salt

**Directions**

1.  Add all the dry ingredients in a bowl then add the egg and water and mix well make sure there are no lumps in your mixture.
2.  Pour the melted butter in the cup you are going to use. You can also use the cup to melt the butter to begin with, but make sure not to over heat the butter; 5 seconds in the microwave should be more than enough. Now swirl the butter around the cup make sure to coat the inside of the cup then pour the butter into the bread mix and combine.
3.  Pour the mix in your cup and microwave for 1.5 minutes. If you are planning on doubling the mix I would suggest using a bigger wider mug or the mix will not cook all the way through. Don't microwave for more than 3 min or the mix will end up hard.
4.  Once you have removed it from the mug, you can then slice it into rounds and place it in the toaster to crisp it up a little.

Servings: 1

**Nutrition Facts** (1 serving)
Calories: 238
Net Carbs: 2.6g
Fat: 19g
Protein: 13g

# Anaheim pepper Gruyere Waffles

**Ingredients**

1 small Anaheim pepper
3 eggs
1/4 cup cream cheese
1/4 cup Gruyere cheese
1 Tbsp. coconut flour
1 tsp. Metamucil powder
1 tsp. baking powder
Salt and pepper to taste

**Directions**

1. In a blender, mix together all ingredients except for the cheese and Anaheim pepper.
2. Once the ingredients are mixed well, add cheese and pepper. Blend well until all ingredients are unit well.
3. Heat your waffle iron; pour on the waffle mix and cook 5-6 minutes.
4. Serve hot.

Servings: 2

Cooking Times
Total Time: 15 minutes

**Nutrition Facts (per serving)**

Calories 223
Fat 17g
Carbs 5,53g
Fiber 0,33g
Sugar 1,56g
Protein 11,6g

# Anchovy, Spinach and Asparagus Omelet

**Ingredients**
2 organic eggs
3/4 cup of spinach
2 oz. anchovy in olive oil
4 marinated asparagus
Celtic Sea salt
Freshly ground black pepper

**Directions**
1. Preheat the oven to 375 F.
2. In the bottom of the baking pan place the anchovy.
3. In a bowl, beat the eggs and pour on top of the fish. Add the spinach and the chopped asparagus on top.
4. Season with salt and pepper to taste.
5. Bake in preheated oven for about 10 minutes.
6. Serve hot.

Servings: 2

Cooking Times
Total Time: 15 minutes

**Nutrition Facts (per serving)**
Calories 83,
Fat 4,91g
Carbs 2,28g
Fiber 0,86g
Sugar 0,23g
Protein 7,7g

# Autumn Pumpkin Bread

**Ingredients**
3 egg whites
1/2 cup coconut milk
1 1/2 cup almond flour
1/2 cup pumpkin puree
2 tsp. baking powder
1 1/2 tsp. Pumpkin pie spice
1/2 tsp. Kosher Salt
coconut oil for greasing

**Directions**
1. Preheat your oven to 350F. Grease a standard bread loaf pan with melted coconut oil.
2. Sift all dry ingredients into a large bowl.
3. In another bowl, add pumpkin puree and coconut milk and mix well. In a separate bowl, beat the egg whites. Fold in egg whites and gently fold into the dough.
4. Spread the dough into the prepared bread pan.
5. Bake the bread for 75 minutes. Once ready, remove bread from the oven and let cool.
6. Slice and serve.

Servings: 8

Cooking Times
Total Time: 1 hour and 25 minutes

**Nutrition Facts (per serving)**
Calories 197
Fat 16,69g
Carbs 8,19g
Fiber 3,31g
Sugar 1,89g
Protein 7,24g

# Batter Coated Cheddar Cheese

**Ingredients**

1 large egg

2 slice Cheddar cheese (3.55 oz.)

1 tsp. ground walnuts

1 tsp. ground flaxseed

2 tsp. almond flour

1 tsp. hemp seeds

1 Tbsp. olive oil

Salt and pepper to taste

**Directions**

1. In a small bowl, whisk an egg together with the salt and pepper.
2. Heat a tablespoon of olive oil in a frying pan, on medium heat.
3. In a separate bowl, mix the ground flaxseed with the ground walnuts, hemp seeds and the almond flour.
4. Coat the cheddar slices with the egg mix, then roll in the dry mix and fry cheese for about 3 minutes on each side. Serve hot.

Servings: 1

Cooking Times
Total Time: 13 minutes

**Nutrition Facts (per serving)**

Calories 509,

Fat 46,19g

Carbs 2,65g

Fiber 0,79g

Protein 21,98g

# Chicken Sausage and Pepper Jack Pie

**Ingredients**

5 egg yolks
1 1/2 chicken sausage
3/4 cup Pepper Jack cheese
1/4 cup coconut flour
2 tsp. lime Juice
1/2 tsp. dried basil
1/4 tsp. baking soda
4 Tbsp. coconut oil
2 Tbsp. coconut water
Kosher salt to taste

**Directions**

1. Preheat oven to 350F.
2. In a frying pan add the sausages and cook on medium high heat 3-4 minutes. Set aside.
3. Measure out the dry ingredients into a bowl.
4. Separate 5 egg yolks from the whites, then discard of the whites.
5. Beat the egg yolks about 4-5 minutes. Add in coconut oil, coconut water, and lime juice. Continue to beat again until smooth and creamy.
6. Mix the wet ingredients into the dry ingredients slowly. At last, add cheese into the batter.
7. Measure out the batter into 2 ramekins. Poke the sausages into the batter.
8. Bake in preheated oven for 25 minutes. Once ready, serve hot.

Servings: 5
Cooking Times
Total Time: 40 minutes

**Nutrition Facts (per serving)**
Calories 294
Fat 24,78g
Carbs 7,66g
Fiber 0,34g
Protein 11g

# Cashew Chocolate & Orange Smoothie

**Ingredients**
1 cup cashew milk
1 handful of arugula leaves
1 Tbsp. chocolate whey protein powder
1/8 tsp. orange extract
Ice cubes

**Directions**
1.  Place all ingredients in your blender and blend until well united and smooth. Add extra ice and serve.

Servings: 1
Cooking Time: 5 minutes

**Nutrition Facts (per serving)**
Calories 44
Fat 1,05g
Carbs 7,1g
Fiber 2,49g
Sugar 4,4g
Protein 3,97g

# Creamy Frappuccino

## Ingredients
1 cup cold coffee
1/3 cup heavy cream
1/4 tsp. xanthan gum
1 tsp. pure vanilla extract
2 Tbsp. Xylitol
6 ice cubes

## Directions
1.  Place all ingredients in your blender. Blend until all unite well and become smooth. Serve.

Servings: 1
Cooking Times: 5 minutes

## Nutrition Facts (per serving)
Calories 287
Fat 29,37g
Carbs 2,74g
Fiber 0g
Protein 1,91g

# Cheesy Boiled Eggs

### Ingredients
3 eggs
2 Tbsp. almond butter, no-stir
2 Tbsp. softened cream cheese
1 tsp. whipping cream
Salt and pepper to taste

### Directions
1. In a small saucepan hard boil the eggs.
2. When ready, wash the eggs with cold water, peel and chop them. Place eggs in a bowl; add in the butter, cream cheese and whipping cream.
3. Mix well and add salt and pepper to taste. Serve.

Servings: 2
Cooking Time: 20 minutes

### Nutrition Facts (per serving)
Calories 212
Fat 19,88g
Carbs 0,75g
Protein 7,74g

# Veggie Scramble

**Ingredients**
4 egg whites
1 egg yolk
2 tbsp. almond milk
1 cup spinach
1 tomato, chopped
½ white onion, chopped
3 fresh basil leaves, chopped
salt and pepper to taste
ghee

**Directions**
1. In a bowl, whisk the egg yolk and whites with the milk. Stir well.
2. Heat the ghee on a pan over medium heat. Add the onions and sauté until fragrant.
3. Throw in the tomato to the pan with the spinach and cook until the spinach is almost wilted.
4. Pour the egg mixture to the spinach and cook until firm or until the egg sets. Stir constantly.
5. Season with salt and pepper.
6. Serve warm

**Nutrition Facts** (per serving)
Calories: 203
Net Carbs: 18g
Fat: 5g
Protein: 20g

# Egg Pesto Scramble

## Ingredients
3 eggs
1 tbsp. pesto sauce
1 tbsp. olive oil
2 tbsp. sour cream

## Directions
1. Whisk the eggs in a bowl and season with salt and pepper.
2. Heat a non-stick pan over low heat. Drizzle with olive oil and pour the eggs. Constantly whisk the eggs while cooking.
3. Add the pesto mixture to the eggs and stir well.
4. Turn off the fire and mix in the sour cream. Combine well.
5. Serve with 1/2 cup mashed avocado.

Servings: 1

## Nutrition Facts (per serving)
Calories: 467
Net Carbs: 3.3g
Fat: 41.5g
Protein: 20.4g

# Cheesy Bread

### Ingredients

125g full-fat cream cheese

1 cup cheddar cheese, grated

3 large eggs

1 tsp. apple cider vinegar

2 cups almond flour

2 tsp. baking powder

1 tsp. mustard powder

1 tsp. salt

### Directions

1. Preheat oven at 375F
2. Combine all the ingredients in a bowl with a hand mixer, except the cheddar cheese.
3. Add the cheddar cheese to the mixture and combine using a spatula or a fork. Be careful not to mush the cheese.
4. Line a bread tin with well-greased baking paper and bake in the oven for 45 minutes.

### Nutrition Facts (per serving)

Calories: 495

Net Carbs: 6.5g

Fat: 9.6g

Protein: 19.7g

# Lemon Cheesecake Breakfast Mousse

## Ingredients

3 tbsp. cream cheese

1 tbsp. lemon juice

50ml heavy cream (look for those with zero carbs)

100ml Yoghurt

1tbsp. Xylitol

1/8 tsp. salt

2 tbsp. whey protein

## Directions

1. Blend cream cheese and lemon juice in a bowl until smooth.
2. Add heavy cream and blend until whipped. Gently add in yoghurt.
3. Taste and adjust sweetener if needed.
4. Serve with ¼ cup berry coulis.

# Berry Breakfast Shake

**Ingredients**
¾ cup mixed berries
1 cup almond milk
1 tbsp. all-natural peanut butter
1 tbsp. protein powder
¼ tsp. cinnamon powder
¼ tsp. ginger, minced

**Directions**
1. Place all the ingredients in a blender and mix until smooth.

Servings: 1

**Nutrition Facts** (per serving)
Calories: 319
Net Carbs: 9g
Fat: 15g
Protein: 28g

# Cacao and Raspberry Pudding

**Ingredients**

1 tbsp. cacao powder

¼ cup raspberry

3 tbsp. chia seeds

1 cup almond milk

1 tsp. agave

**Directions**

2. In a small bowl, combine the almond milk and cacao powder. Stir well.
3. Add the chia seeds to the bowl and let it rest for 5 minutes.
4. Using a fork, fluff the chia and cacao mixture and then place in the fridge to chill for at least 30 minutes.
5. Serve with raspberries and a drizzle of agave on top

# Coco and Blueberry Smoothie

**Ingredients**
½ cup blueberries
½ cup coconut cream
1 tbsp. coconut oil
½ cup almond milk, vanilla flavor
3 ice cubes

**Directions**
1. Place all the ingredients in a blender and mix until you achieve a smooth consistency.

Servings: 2

**Nutrition info for one serving:**
Calories 295
Fat 24g
Protein 13g
Carbs 6g
Fibre 1g

# Creamy Chocolate Milk

### Ingredients

16 ounces unsweetened almond milk

1 teaspoon xylitol

4 ounces heavy cream

1 scoop Whey Chocolate Isolate powder

1/2 cup crushed ice (optional: add if you like a thick drink, but the flavour will be less intense.)

### Directions

1.   Put all ingredients in blender and blend until smooth.

Servings: 2

### Nutrition info for one serving:

Calories 292

Fat 25g

Protein 15g

Carbs 5g

# Blueberry Almond Smoothie

### Ingredients
16 ounces unsweetened almond milk
1 teaspoon xylitol
4 ounces heavy cream
1/4 cup frozen unsweetened blueberries
1 scoop Whey Vanilla protein powder

### Directions
1. Put all ingredients in blender and blend until smooth.
2. Add a little water if it becomes too thick.
3. Measure those blueberries as they add more carbs.

Servings: 2

### Nutrition info for one serving:
Calories 302
Fat 25g
Protein 15g
Carbs 6g
Fibre 1g

# Mozzarella, Red Pepper & Bacon Frittata

**Ingredients**

Olive oil (1 tablespoon)

Parsley (2 tablespoons, chopped)

Mozzarella cheese (4 oz., cubed)

Bell pepper (1, red, chopped)

Heavy cream (1/4 cup)

Bacon (7 slices)

Bella mushrooms (4 caps, large)

Basil (1/2 cup, chopped)

Goat cheese (2 oz., grated)

Eggs (9)

Parmesan cheese (1/4 cup, grated)

Salt & Black pepper

**Directions**

1. Set oven to 350 F.
2. Chop red pepper, bacon, basil and mushroom. Slice mozzarella into cubes and put aside.
3. Heat olive oil in a skillet until it slightly smokes then add bacon and cook for 5 minutes until browned.
4. Add red pepper and cook for 2 minutes until soft. While pepper cooks, add cream, parmesan cheese, eggs and black pepper to a bowl and whisk to combine.
5. Add mushrooms to pot, stir and cook for 5 minutes until soaked in fat. Add basil, cook for 1 minute then add mozzarella.
6. Put in egg mixture and use spoon to move ingredients around so that the egg gets on the bottom of pan.
7. Top with goat cheese and place in oven for 8 minutes then broil for 6 minutes.
8. Use knife to pry frittata edges from pan and place on a plate and slice. Serve.

Servings: 6

**Nutrition Facts (per serving)**

Calories 408

Net Carbs 2.4g

Fats 31.2g

Protein 19.2g

Fiber 0.8g

# Rosemary, Sausage & Cheese Pies

**Ingredients**

Cheddar cheese (3/4 cup, grated)
Coconut oil (1/4 cup)
Egg yolks (5)
Rosemary (1/2 teaspoon)
Baking soda (1/4 teaspoon)
Chicken sausage (1 ½)
Coconut flour (1/4 cup)
Coconut milk (2 tablespoons)
Lemon juice (2 teaspoons)
Cayenne pepper (1/4 teaspoon)
Kosher salt (1/8 teaspoon)

**Directions**

1. Set oven to 350 F.
2. Chop sausage, heat skillet and cook sausage. While sausages cook combine all dry ingredients in a bowl. In another bowl combine lemon juice, oil and coconut milk. Add liquids to dry mixture and add ½ cup of cheese; fold to combine and put into 2 ramekins.
3. Add cooked sausages to batter and use spoon to push into mixture.
4. Bake for 25 minutes until golden on top. Top with leftover cheese and broil for 4 minutes.
5. Serve warm.

Servings: 2

**Nutrition Facts (per serving)**

Calories 711
Net Carbs 5.8g
Fats 65.3g
Protein 34.3g
Fiber 11.5g

# Kale Sausage Omelet Pie

**Ingredients**
10 eggs
1 1/2 cup Mahón cheese (or Cheddar)
3 chicken sausages
3 cups raw chopped Kale leaves
2 1/2 cup mushrooms, chopped
1 Tbsp. garlic powder
2 tsp. hot sauce
1/2 tsp. black pepper and celery seed
salt and pepper to taste

**Directions**
1. Preheat oven to 400F.
2. Chop up your sausage and mushroom thin and place them in a cast iron skillet. Cook on a medium-high heat for 2-3 minutes.
3. While the sausages are cooking, chop your spinach up. Add in a skillet the mushrooms and spinach.
4. In a meanwhile, in a bowl mix eggs with black pepper and celery seed, hot sauce, and spices. Scramble them well.
5. Mix your sausages, spinach, and mushrooms so that the spinach can wilt fully. Add salt and pepper to taste.
6. Finally, add the cheese to the top.
7. Pour your eggs over the mixture and mix everything well.
8. Stir the mixture for a few seconds, and then put your cast iron skillet in the oven. Bake for 10-12 minutes, and then broil the top for 3-4 minutes.
9. Let cool for a while, cut into 8 slices and serve hot.

Servings: 8
Cooking Time: 25 minutes

**Nutrition Facts (per serving)**
Calories 266
Fat 17,76g
Carbs 7,67g
Fiber 0,92g
Protein 19,37g

# Bacon, Scallions & Monterey Omelet

**Ingredients**

2 eggs
2 slices cooked bacon
1/4 cup scallions, chopped
1/4 cup Monterey jack cheese
salt and pepper to taste
1 tsp. lard

**Directions**

1. In a frying pan heat lard in on medium-low heat. Add the eggs, scallions and salt and pepper to taste.
2. Cook for 1-2 minutes; add the bacon and sauté 30 - 45 seconds longer. Turn the heat off on the stove.
3. On top of the bacon place a cheese. Then, take two edges of the omelet and fold them onto the cheese. Hold the edges there for a moment as the cheese has to partially melt. Make the same with the other egg and let cook in a warm pan for a while.
4. Serve hot.

Servings: 2
Cooking Time: 15 minutes

**Nutrition Facts (per serving)**

Calories 321
Fat 28,31g
Carbs 1,62g
Fiber 0,33g
Protein 14,37g

# Bacon, Avocado & Smoked Turkey Muffins

**Ingredients**

5 eggs
6 slices smoked turkey bacon
1/2 cup almond flour
2 medium Avocados
1/2 cup Cheddar cheese
1 1/2 cup coconut milk
3 spring onions
1 tsp. minced garlic
2 tsp. dried parsley
1/4 tsp. red chili powder
1 1/2 Tbsp. lemon juice
1/4 cup flaxseed
1 1/2 Tbsp. Metamucil powder
1 tsp. baking powder
2 Tbsp. butter
salt & pepper to taste

**Directions**

1. Preheat oven to 350F.
2. In a frying pan over medium-low heat, cook the bacon with the butter until crisp. Add the spring onions, cheese, and baking powder.
3. In a bowl, mix together coconut milk, eggs, Metamucil powder, almond flour, flax, spices and lemon juice. Switch off the heat and let cool. Then, crumble the bacon and add all of the fat to the egg mixture. Clean and chop avocado and fold into the mixture.
4. Measure out batter into a cupcake tray that's been sprayed or greased with nonstick spray and bake for 25-26 minutes.
5. Once ready, let cool and serve hot or cold.

Servings: 16
Cooking Time: 40 minutes
**Nutrition Facts (per serving)**
Calories 184
Fat 16,4g
Carbs 5,51g
Fiber 2,7g
Protein 5,89g

# Cream Cheese Pancakes

### Ingredients
2 eggs
1/4 cup cream cheese
1 Tbsp. coconut flour
1 tsp. ground ginger
1/2 cup liquid Stevia
coconut oil
sugar-free maple syrup

### Directions
1.  In a deep bowl, beat together all of the ingredients until smooth.
2.  Heat up a frying skillet with oil on medium-high. Ladle the batter and pour in hot oil.
3.  Cook on one side and then flip. Top with a sugar-free maple syrup and serve.

Servings: 16
Cooking Time: 15 minutes

### Nutrition Facts (per serving)
Calories 170, 78
Fat 13,71g
Carbs 4,39g
Fiber 0,14g
Protein 6,9g

# Adorable Pumpkin Flaxseed Muffins

## Ingredients

1 egg

1 1/4 cup flaxseeds (ground)

1 cup  pumpkin puree

1 Tbs pumpkin pie spice

2 Tbs coconut oil

1/2 cup sweetener of your choice

1 tsp. baking powder

2 tsp. cinnamon

1/2 tsp. apple cider vinegar

1/2 tsp. vanilla extract

salt to taste

## Directions

1. Preheat your oven to 360°F.
2. First, grind the flaxseeds for several seconds.
3. Put together all the dry ingredients and stir.
4. Then, add your pumpkin puree and mix to combine.
5. Add the vanilla extract and the pumpkin spice.
6. Add in coconut oil, egg and apple vinegar. Add sweetener of your choice and stir again.
7. Add a heaping tablespoon of batter to each lined muffin or cupcake and top with some pumpkin seeds.
8. Bake for about 18 - 20 minutes. Serve hot.

Servings: 10

## Cooking Times

Total Time: 20 minutes

## Nutrition Facts (per serving)

Carbs: 3g

Fiber: 1g

Protein: 1g

Fat: 5.34g

Calories: 43

# Baked Ham and Kale Scrambled Eggs

**Ingredients**
5 ounces ham diced
2 medium eggs
1 green onion, finely chopped
1/2 cups kale leaves, chopped
1 garlic clove, crushed
1 green chilli, finely chopped
4 ready-roasted peppers
pinch cayenne pepper
1 Tbsp. olive oil
1/2 can water

**Directions**
1. Heat oven to 360F.
2. Heat the oil in a small ovenproof frying pan. Add green onion and cook for 4-5 mins until softened.
3. Stir in the garlic and chilli, and cook for a couple mins more.
4. Add the 1/2 cup water. Season well and stir through the ready-roasted peppers and ham. Bring to a simmer and cook for 10 mins.
5. Add the kale, stirring through to wilt.
6. In a small bowl, beat the eggs with a pinch of cayenne and pour in frying pan together with other ingredients.
7. Transfer the frying pan to the oven & bake for 10 mins. Serve hot.

Servings: 2

**Cooking Times**
Preparation Time: 10 minutes
Cooking Time: 30 minutes
Total Time: 2 hours and 20 minutes

**Nutrition Facts (per serving)**
Carbs: 3,8g
Fiber: 0,8g
Protein: 22g
Fat: 15,74g
Calories: 251

# Bell Pepper and Ham Omelet

## Ingredients
4 large eggs
1 cup green pepper (chopped)
1/4 lb ham, cooked and diced
1 green onion, diced
1 tsp. coconut oil
salt and freshly ground pepper to taste

## Directions
1. Wash and chop vegetables. Set aside.
2. Into a small bowl beat the eggs. Set aside.
3. Heat non-stick skillet over medium heat and add coconut oil. Pour half of the beaten eggs into the skillet.
4. When the egg has partially set, add half of the vegetables and ham to one half of the omelet and continue to cook until the egg is almost fully set.
5. Fold the empty half over top of the ham and veggies using a spatula.
6. Cook for 2 minutes more and then serve.
7. Serve hot.

Servings: 2

## Nutrition Facts (per serving)
Carbs: 6,8g
Protein: 21,88g
Fat: 12g
Calories: 225,76

# Chia Flour Pancakes

**Ingredients**
1 cup Chia flour
2 tsp. sweetener of your choice
1 egg, beaten
1 Tbsp. coconut butter or oil
1/2 cup coconut milk (canned)

**Directions**
1. In a medium bowl, combine the flour and sugar. Add the egg, milk and coconut butter. Mix well until make a smooth batter.
2. Grease a non-stick skillet and heat over medium-high heat. Drop a heaping tablespoon of batter onto the hot surface.
3. When bubbles form on the surface of the scones, use a spatula to turn them and then cook about 2 minutes per side.
4. Serve hot.

Servings: 6
Cooking Time: 15 minutes

**Nutrition Facts (per serving)**
Carbs: 4,65g
Protein: 2,46g
Fat: 3,5g
Calories: 59

# Choco Moko Chia Porridge

**Ingredients**

3 Tbs Chia Seeds
1 cup almond milk, unsweetened
2 tsp. cocoa powder
1/4 cup raspberries -fresh or frozen
2 Tbsp. almond, ground
Sweetener of your choice (optional)

**Directions**

1. Mix and stir the almond milk and the cocoa powder together.
2. Add the Chia Seeds in the mixture.
3. Mix well with a fork.
4. Place the mixture in a fridge for 30 minutes.
5. Serve with raspberries and ground almonds on the top. (optional)

Servings: 2
Inactive Time: 30 minutes. Cooking Time: 5 minutes

**Nutrition Facts (per serving)**

Carbs: 15,2g
Fiber: 11,28g
Protein: 5,47g
Fat: 9,62g
Calories: 150,1

# Coffee Flaxseed Dream Breakfast

**Ingredients**

3 Tbsp. flaxseed, ground

1/2 cup strong black coffee, unsweetened

2 1/2 Tbsp. coconut flakes, unsweetened

1 Tbsp. coconut oil, melted

Sweetener of your choice to taste

1/2 cup water (optional)

**Directions**

1. In a bowl, combine the flaxseed and the coconut flakes.
2. Add the melted coconut oil, then pour the hot coffee over it and mix.
3. If it is too thick, add a little water.
4. At the end, add the sweetener of your choice to taste.
5. Ready! Enjoy!!

Servings: 1

**Nutrition Facts (per serving)**

Carbs: 1,52

Fiber: 0,9g

Protein: 1,48g

Fat: 22,1

Calories: 246,43

# Crimini Mushroom with Boiled Eggs Breakfast

## Ingredients
14 Crimini mushroom, finely chopped
8 large eggs, hard-boiled, chopped
6 slices  bacon or pancetta
1 spring onion, diced
Salt and ground black pepper to taste

## Directions
1. In a frying pan cook bacon. Reserve a bacon fat in the pan. Chop up bacon pieces and set aside.
2. In a deep saucepan, hard-boil the eggs. When ready, wah, clean, shell and chop into bite-size pieces.
3. In a frying pan cook the spring onion with remaining bacon fat over medium-high heat.
4. Add the Crimini mushrooms and sauté another 5-6 minutes.
5. Blend the eggs, bacon and cook together. Adjust salt and ground black pepper to taste.
6. Serve.

Servings: 6
Cooking Time: 20 minutes

## Nutrition Facts (per serving)
Carbs: 2,43g
Fiber: 1,5g
Protein: 11,32
Fat: 13
Calories: 176

# Egg Whites and Spinach Omelet

**Ingredients**
5 egg whites
2 Tbsp. almond milk
1 zucchini, shredded
1 cup spinach leaves, fresh
2 Tbs spring onion, chopped
2 cloves garlic
Olive oil
Basil leaves, fresh, chopped
Salt and ground black pepper to taste

**Directions**
1. Wash and chop the vegetables
2. In a bowl, beat the egg whites and the almond milk.
3. In a greased frying pan with olive oil, cook the vegetables (spinach, zucchini, spring onion) just for one to two minutes.
4. Put the vegetables on the side, grease the pan again with olive oil and pour the eggs. Cook until the eggs are firm. Add the vegetables on one side and cook for two minutes more. Adjust salt and pepper to taste.
5. Decorate with basil leaves and serve.

Servings: 2

**Cooking Times**
Total Time: 15 minutes

**Nutrition Facts (per serving)**
Carbs: 5,78g
Fiber: 1,58g
Protein: 11,08g
Fat: 1,56g
Calories: 70,8

# Fast Protein and Peanut-Butter Pancakes

**Ingredients**

1 scoop of low-carb protein powder

2 eggs

2 Tbsp. of natural peanut butter

2 Tbsp. flaxseed

2 Tbsp. water

olive oil for greasing

**Directions**

1. In a bowl, mix protein powder, eggs, peanut butter, water and flaxseeds.
2. Grease with olive oil and heat a large non-stick frying pan over medium heat.
3. Ladle a batter mixture and cook for 2 minutes per side or until bubbles appear on surface. Transfer to a plate.
4. Serve hot.

Servings: 1

Cooking Time: 15 minutes

**Nutrition Facts (per serving)**

Carbs: 13,78g

Fiber: 8,48g

Protein: 17,8g

Fat: 23,59g

Calories: 406,41

# Guacamole Bacon and Eggs Breakfast

**Ingredients**

4 slices  bacon or pancetta

2 Tbsp. heavy cream

2 Tbsp.  avocado oil

4 eggs

salt and pepper to taste

**Directions**

1.  In a bowl, beat eggs with heavy cream and salt and ground pepper to taste.
2.  Pour egg mixture over bacon and cook for 2-3 minutes.
3.  Flip bacon and eggs on other side and cook for 1 minute more.
4.  Serve and enjoy!

Servings: 4

Cooking Time: 13 minutes

**Nutrition Facts (per serving)**

Carbs: 0,66g

Fiber: 0g

Protein: 9,28g

Fat: 22,43g

Calories: 292

# Hemp Muffins with Walnuts

## Ingredients

2 1/2 cup Hemp flour

1 1/2 cup walnuts, chopped

1/2 cup sweetener of your choice

4 Tbsp. extra-virgin olive oil

1 tsp. vanilla extract

2 tsp. baking powder

1 tsp. baking soda

## Directions

1. Preheat oven to 345F.
2. In a small bowl whisk olive oil, sweetener of your choice and vanilla.
3. In a separate bowl, combine hemp flour, baking powder and baking soda. Add in chopped walnuts and toss to coat.
4. Add olive oil mixture to the flour mixture and stir slightly.
5. Spoon a batter into 12 muffin cups, filling 3/4 full.
6. Bake 18 - 20 minutes. Allow to cool 10 minutes in the muffin pan, then turn out onto a wire rack to cool completely. Serve.

Servings: 12

Cooking Time: 30 minutes

## Nutrition Facts (per serving)

Carbs: 25,18g

Fiber: 4,43g

Protein: 7,75g

Fat: 16,45g

Calories: 270

# Baked Pancetta and Eggs

**Ingredients**
6 slices Pancetta, crumbled
8 eggs
3/4 cup Cheddar cheese, grated
3/4 cup heavy cream
salt and pepper to taste
olive oil for greasing

**Directions**
1. Preheat the oven to 350 degrees F. Grease a big baking dish with olive oil.
2. In a bowl, beat the eggs with shredded Cheddar cheese and cream, and season with salt and pepper to taste.
3. Crumble Pancetta evenly over the egg mixture. Put the baking dish in a preheated oven.
4. Bake for 15 minutes.
5. Serve immediately.

Servings: 6
Cooking Times: 20 minutes

**Nutrition Facts (per serving)**
Carbs: 1,49g
Fiber: 0g
Protein: 12,5g
Fat: 22,03g
Calories: 254,89

# Bilberry Coconut Mush

**Ingredients**
1/4 cup coconut flour
1 cup coconut milk
1/4 cup ground flaxseed
1 tsp. vanilla extract
1 tsp. cinnamon
Liquid sweetener of your choice

**Toppings**
1 cup bilberries
2 Tbs shaved coconut
2 Tbs pumpkin seeds

**Directions**
1. In a saucepan heat the coconut milk. Add in coconut flour, cinnamon and flaxseed and whisk.
2. Add in vanilla extract and liquid sweetener of your choice. Cook for 10 minutes stirring constantly. Remove from heat and let cook for 2-3 minutes.
3. Decorate with fresh bilberries, pumpkin seeds and shaved coconut to taste.

Servings: 2

**Cooking Times**
Total Time: 5 minutes

**Nutrition Facts (per serving)**
Carbs: 16,4g
Fiber: 1,69
Protein: 2,86g
Fat: 22,4f
Calories:445

# Boiled Eggs with Mascarpone and Bacon

**Ingredients**
2 large eggs
2 Tbsp. Mascarpone cheese
2 Tbs crumbled bacon
1 Tbs coconut butter
salt and pepper to taste

**Directions**
1. Hard boil the eggs; bring water to a boil over medium-high heat, then cover, remove from the heat and set aside for 10 minutes.
2. Wash, peel and chop boiled eggs and place them in a large bowl.
3. Add the butter and the Mascarpone cheese, mix well. Adjust salt and pepper to taste.
4. Serve.

Servings: 2
Cooking Time: 15 minutes

**Nutrition Facts (per serving)**
Carbs: 0,91g
 Fiber: 0g
Protein: 11,1g
Fat: 22,84g
Calories: 328,34

# Flax-Almond Coated Cheddar

**Ingredients**

4 oz Cheddar cheese, 2 slices
1 large egg
1 tsp. almond flour or ground almonds
1 Tbsp. flaxseed, ground
1 tsp. hemp seeds
1 Tbsp. Olive oil
Salt and pepper to taste

**Directions**

1. In a non-stick frying pan heat a tablespoon of olive oil.
2. In a bowl, combine the almond flour, the ground flaxseed and the hemp seeds.
3. In a separate bowl, beat an egg together with the salt and pepper.
4. Coat the cheddar slices first with the egg mix and then with the dry mix. Fry cheese for about 3 minutes on each side. Serve hot.

Servings: 2
Cooking Time: 15 minutes

**Nutrition Facts (per serving)**

Carbs: 4,28g
Fiber: 2,83g
Protein: 17,91g
Fat: 22,37g
Calories: 358,62

# French Almond Toast

**Ingredients**
4 eggs
1/4 cup coconut milk
2 Tbsp. coconut oil (melted)
6 slices almond bread
2 tsp. sweetener of your choice (optional)
1/2 tsp. cinnamon powder
1 tsp. organic vanilla extract
salt and pepper (per taste)

**Directions**
1. Whisk coconut milk, sweetener of your choice, eggs, organic vanilla extract, salt and cinnamon.
2. Soak each slice of almond bread (or any gluten free vegan Hemp & Seed bread) in egg mixture.
3. In a frying pan, heat the coconut oil over high heat; cook each slice of bread three minutes or until golden. Transfer toast to the plate lined with paper.
4. Serve hot.

Servings: 6

**Nutrition Facts (per serving)**
Carbs: 11,13g
Fiber: 0,57g
Protein: 6,56g
Fat: 10,2g
Calories: 162,6

# Pork and Sage Breakfast Burgers

**Ingredients**

1 lb ground pork

2 Tbsp. fresh sage, chopped

1 tsp. garlic powder

1 tsp. cayenne pepper

salt and pepper to taste

2 Tbsp. granular sweetener of your choice

olive oil for greasing

**Directions**

1. In a large bowl, combine all ingredients except olive oil. Use hands to mix thoroughly.
2. Form into 8 evenly burgers.
3. Grease with olive oil your large frying pan over medium heat.
4. Add burger and cook about 3 to 4 minutes per side.
5. Ready. Serve and enjoy!!

Servings: 4

Cooking Time: 15 minutes

**Nutrition Facts (per serving)**

Carbs: 0,78g

Fiber: 0,44g

Protein: 19,29g

Fat: 22,17g

Calories: 302,21

# Quick & Easy Flax "Muffins"

### Ingredients
4 Tbsp. ground flax meal
1 egg
1 Tbs of heavy whipping cream
1 tsp. organic vanilla extract
2 tsp. sweetener of your choice
1 pinch salt
coconut butter
cocoa powder (optional)

### Directions
1.  Mix all ingredients in a microwave safe bowl; stir to combine well.
2.  Place a bit of coconut butter on the top. Microwave for one and a half minutes.
3.  If you want, you can add a splash of unsweetened cocoa powder.
4.  Ready! Serve! Enjoy!

Servings: 1

### Cooking Times
Total Time: 5 minutes

### Nutrition Facts (per serving)
Carbs: 10,24g
Fiber: 1,36g
Protein: 8,21g
Fat: 8,4g
Calories: 160,51

# Millet Gingerbread Mash

**Ingredients**

1 cup millet flour (or any kind of whole grain flour)

4 cups water

1/2 tsp. ground ginger

1/4 tsp. ground allspice

1/8 tsp. ground nutmeg

1/4 tsp. ground cardamom

1/4 tsp. ground coriander

1 1/2 Tbs ground cinnamon

1 tsp. ground cloves

sweetener of your choice (optional)

**Directions**

1. In a medium saucepan bring water to boiling and cook the millet flour to package direction. Add in all spices together and stir.
2. Reduce heat and simmer, uncovered, for 5 minutes, stirring occasionally.
3. When cooked, add sweetener to taste.

Servings: 6

**Nutrition Facts (per serving)**

Carbs: 11,13g

Fiber: 2,6g

Protein: 1,9g

Fat: 2.82g

Calories: 58,18

# Scrambled Eggs with Bacon and Gouda Cheese

**Ingredients**
4 strips cooked bacon
4 eggs
2 1/2 Tbsp. olive oil
1/4 cup softened cream cheese
1/4 cup shredded Gouda cheese
garlic and onion powder
black or white pepper

**Directions**
1. In a frying pan heat some olive oil and fry bacon slices until crisp
   .
2. In a small bowl beat the eggs with onion and garlic powder, cream cheese and Gouda shredded cheese. Season with salt and pepper to taste.
3. Pour egg mixture over bacon slices and cook for 3-4 minutes. Serve and enjoy!

Servings: 4
Cooking Time: 15 minutes

**Nutrition Facts (per serving)**
Carbs: 1,47g
Fiber: 0g
Protein: 14,44g
Fat: 25,94g
Calories: 380,72

# Beet Cucumber Smoothie

## Ingredients

1 cup spinach leaves

2 cups cucumber (peeled, seeded and chopped)

1/2 cup carrot chopped

1/2 cup fresh beetroot

3/4 cup heavy (whipping) cream

4 tsp. sweetener of your choice (optional)

Handful of ground almonds

1 cup ice cubes

1 cup water

## Directions

1. Place all ingredients in a blender.
2. Pulse until smooth.
3. Serve immediately.

Servings: 4

Cooking Time: 5 minutes

## Nutrition Facts (per serving)

Carbs: 6,19g

Protein: 1,66g

Fat: 12.99g

Calories: 137,91

# Cilantro and Ginger Smoothie

**Ingredients**

1/2 cup fresh cilantro (chopped)
2 inch ginger, fresh
1 cucumber
2 Tbsp. chia seeds
1/2 cup spinach, fresh
1 Tbsp. almond butter
Handful of ground almond
1 lime (or lemon)
2 cups water

**Directions**

1.  Blend spinach, coriander and water until smooth.
2.  Add the remaining fruits and blend again.

Servings: 3
Cooking Time: 5 minutes

**Nutrition Facts (per serving)**

Carbs: 11,98g
Fiber: 6,88g
Protein:
Fat: 6.92g
Calories: 102,72

# Green Coconut Smoothie

### Ingredients
1 cup coconut milk
1 green apple, cored and chopped
1 cup spinach
1 cucumber
2 Tbsp. shaved coconut
1/2 cup water
ice cubes (if needed)

### Directions
1. Put all ingredients and ice in a blender; pulse until smooth.
2. Serve immediately.

Servings: 2
Cooking Time: 5 minutes

### Nutrition Facts (per serving)
Carbs: 18,11g
Fiber: 4g
Protein: 2,88g
Fat: 16,56g
Calories: 216,57

# Green Devil Smoothie

**Ingredients**
3 cup kale, fresh
1/2 cup coconut yogurt
1/2 cup broccoli, florets
2 celery stalk, chopped
2 cup water
1 Tbsp. lemon juice
ice cubes (if needed)

**Directions**
1.  Blend all ingredients together until smooth and slightly frothy.

Servings: 2
Cooking Time: 10 minutes

**Nutrition Facts (per serving)**
Carbs: 16,42g
Fiber: 6,18g
Protein: 4,09g
Fat: 4,98g
Calories: 117,09

# Green Dream Smoothie

**Ingredients**

1 cup raw cucumber, peeled and sliced

4 cups water

1 cup romaine lettuce

1 cup Haas avocado

2 Tbsp. fresh basil

sweetener of your choice (optional)

handful of walnuts

2 Tbsp. fresh parsley

1 Tbsp. fresh ginger grated

ice cubes (optional)

**Directions**

1. In a blender, combine all of the ingredients and puls until smooth.
2. Add ice if used. Serve cold.

Servings: 4

**Nutrition Facts (per serving)**

Carbs: 4,1g

Protein: 1,1g

Fat: 3,89g

Calories: 50,62

# Green Pistachio Smoothie

### Ingredients
2 celery stem with leaves
1 cup spinach leaves, roughly chopped
1/2 cup pistachio nuts (unsalted)
1/2 avocado, chopped
1/2 cup lime, juice
1 Tbsp. Hemp seeds
1 Tbsp. soaked almonds
1 cup coconut water or water
ice cubes (optional)

### Directions
1. Mix all ingredients in a blender with a few ice cubes until smooth.

Servings: 2
Cooking Time: 10 minutes

### Nutrition Facts (per serving)
Carbs: 14,4g
Fiber: 9,8g
Protein: 11,08g
Fat: 17,88g
Calories: 349,55

# Lime Peppermint Smoothie

**Ingredients**
1/4 cup fresh mint leaves
1/4 cup lime juice
1/2 cup cucumber, chopped
1 Tbsp. fresh basil leaves, chopped
1 tsp. chia seed (optional)
Handful of chia seeds
3 tsp. zest of limes
sweetener of your choice to taste
1 cup water, divided
Ice as needed

**Directions**
1. Place all ingredients in a blender or food processor. Pulse until smooth well.
2. Fill glasses with ice, pour the limeade into each glass, and enjoy!

Servings: 4

**Cooking Times**
Total Time: 5 minutes

**Nutrition Facts (per serving)**
Carbs: 4,49g
Fiber: 1,98g
Protein: 0,84g
Fat: 1,16g
Calories: 28,11

# Red Grapefruit Kale Smoothies

### Ingredients
2 cups Cantaloupe

1/4 cup fresh strawberries

8 oz coconut yogurt

2 cups kale leaves, chopped

2 Tbsp. sweetener of your taste

1 Ice as needed

1 cup water

### Directions
1. Clean the grapefruit and remove the seeds.
2. Combine all ingredients in an electric blender and whirl until smooth. Add ice if used and serve.

Servings: 4

Cooking Time: 10 minutes

### Nutrition Facts (per serving)
Carbs: 14g

Fiber: 7,23g

Protein: 4,42g

Fat: 11,57g

Calories: 260,74

# Simple Avocado Smoothie

**Ingredients**

2.6 oz avocado

2 cup water

2 tsp. chia seeds

0.5 oz fresh spinach

2 fl oz heavy whipping cream

1 tsp. vanilla extract, unsweetened

1 Tbsp. extra virgin coconut oil

liquid Stevia extract

few ice cubes

**Directions**

1. First, bisect the avocado. Carefully remove the seed.
2. In a blender, put all ingredients, sweetener and the ice (if used) and beat until smooth. Serve.

Servings: 2

Cooking Time: 10 minutes

**Nutrition Facts (per serving)**

Carbs: 4,46g

Protein: 1,66g

Fat: 23,63g

Calories: 226,44

# Vanilla Protein Smoothie

### Ingredients
1 cup baby spinach
5 Tbsp. of heavy cream
3 Tbsp. organic nut butter of your choice
1/2 cup vanilla protein powder
3 Tbsp. sweetener of your choice
1 cup of water
Ice cubes

### Directions
1. Place all ingredients in a blender and pulse until smooth well.
2. Serve with ice cubes (optional).

Servings: 2
Cooking Time: 5 minutes

### Nutrition Facts (per serving)
Carbs: 11,88g
Fiber: 4,63g
Protein: 8,41g
Fat: 21,79g
Calories: 256,18

# Ail Creamy Brussels Sprouts

**Ingredients**
10 Brussels sprouts
4 cloves garlic
1/4 cup cream cheese
2 Tbsp. extra virgin olive oil
1 tsp. Balsamic vinegar
salt and pepper to taste

**Directions**
1. Clean the Brussels Sprouts discarding the first leaves and cut into julienne strips.
2. Peel and chop the garlic cloves.
3. In a frying pan, heat the olive oil and saute the Brussels Sprouts and garlic,
4. When the garlic and sprouts are tender, turn off the heat and add the cheese. Let sit for a couple of minutes.
5. Transfer to plate and enjoy!

Servings: 1
Cooking Time: 15 minutes

**Nutrition Facts (per serving)**
Carbs: 16,99g
Fiber: 6,22g
Protein: 9,27g
Fat: 12,55g
Calories: 223,26

# Baked Broccoli with Mushrooms and Parmesan

### Ingredients
4 cups broccoli
2 cups mushrooms (chopped fine)
2 Tbsp. minced garlic
1/2 tsp. dried oregano
3 Tbsp. grated Parmesan
salt and ground black pepper to taste

### Directions
1.  Preheat oven to 300F. Line a baking sheet with parchment paper.
2.  Wash and slice broccoli into florets. In a bowl, toss broccoli and finely chopped mushrooms in olive oil. Season with dried oregano, salt and pepper to taste.
3.  Spread all vegetables evenly over the prepared baking pan. Bake for 20-25 minutes until the broccoli is browned.
4.  When done, leave to cool 5 minutes, sprinkle with Parmesan cheese and serve.

Servings: 2

### Cooking Times
Total Time: 35 minutes

### Nutrition Facts (per serving)
Carbs: 16,22g
Fiber: 3,33g
Protein: 12,16g
Fat: 3,51g
Calories: 138,26

# Baked Buckwheat Pancakes with Hazelnuts

**Ingredients**
1/2 cup buckwheat flour
3 eggs
1/2 cup coconut cream
1 vanilla bean (seeds only)
1 pinch of salt
3 Tbsp. olive oil
Liquid sweetener of your choice
hazelnuts

**Directions**
1. Preheat oven to 400F degrees.
2. Grease an oval baking pan.
3. In a large bowl, add eggs, milk, flour, vanilla and salt. Mix the ingredients until the mixture become homogeneous.
4. Pour batter in prepared oval baking pan evenly. Bake for 15-20 minutes.
5. Remove the pancake from the pan and serve with sweetener of your taste and hazelnuts.

Servings: 2

**Cooking Times**
Total Time: 30 minutes

**Nutrition Facts (per serving)**
Carbs: 17,46g
Fiber: 3g
Protein: 14,4g
Fat: 22,66g
Calories: 390,07

# Baked Parmesan-Almond Zucchini

**Ingredients**
2 zucchinis, thinly sliced to about 1-inch thick rounds
3 large eggs, beaten
1 cup almond flour
1 cup almonds, ground
1 cup grated Parmesan cheese
1 tsp. dried oregano
salt and pepper

**Directions**
1. Preheat oven to 400 F degrees. Line a large baking sheet with parchment paper.
2. Wash, clean and slice zucchinis. Salt from all sides and let dry on a paper towel. Set aside.
3. In a plate, combine ground almond, Parmesan cheese, oregano and season with salt and pepper to taste and oregano; set aside.
4. In another shallow plate add the almond flour.
5. In a third plate beat eggs, with salt and pepper.
6. Start dredging zucchini rounds in flour, dip into eggs, then dredge in almond mixture, pressing to coat. Place zucchini slices on prepared baking sheet.
7. Bake for 20 to 30 minutes, or until the zucchini rounds are golden and crispy.
8. Serve hot.

Servings: 6

**Cooking Times**
Preparation Time: 15 minutes
Cooking Time: 25 minutes

**Nutrition Facts (per serving)**
Carbs: 16,36g
Dietary Fiber: 3,28g
Protein: 12,12g
Fat: 17,49g
Calories: 288

114

# Double Cheese Artichoke Dip

**Ingredients**
2 cup artichoke hearts, chopped
16 oz shredded Mozzarella cheese
1 cup grated Parmesan cheese
1 cup heavy (whipping) cream
1 cup green onion, grated

**Directions**
1. Mix all ingredients together and put in a Slow Cooker.
2. Cook on HIGH mode for about one hour.
3. Sprinkle with chopped green onion, if desired.

Servings: 12

**Cooking Times**
Total Time: 1 hour

**Nutrition Facts (per serving)**
Carbs: 10,44g
Fiber: 1,74g
Protein: 13,67g
Total Fat: 15g
Calories: 227

# Easy Slow Cooker Artichokes

**Ingredients**
4 artichokes
3 Tbsp. lemon juice
2 Tbsp. coconut butter, melted
1 tsp. salt and ground black pepper to taste
water

**Directions**
1. Wash and trim artichokes.
2. Start by pulling off the outermost leaves until you get down to the lighter yellow leaves.
3. Then, using a serrated knife, cut off the top third or so of the artichoke.
4. With the same serrated knife, trim the very bottom of the stem.
5. Mix together salt, melted coconut butter and lemon juice and pour over artichokes.
6. Pour in water to cover 3 of artichokes. Cover and cook on LOW 8-10 hours or on HIGH 2-4 hours.
7. Serve and enjoy!

Servings: 4

**Cooking Times**
Total Time: 2 hours and 10 minutes

**Nutrition Facts (per serving)**
Carbs: 14,52g
Fiber: 6,95g
Protein: 4,29g
Fat: 6,98g
Calories: 113

# Eggs with Motley Peppers and Zucchini

## Ingredients

6 eggs

2 zucchini, diced

1 spring onion, chopped

1 green pepper, finely diced

1 yellow pepper, finely diced

1 red pepper, finely diced

3 Tbsp. coconut oil (melted)

salt and fresh ground black pepper to taste

## Directions

1. In a non-stick frying skillet, heat 2 Tbsp. olive oil in a pan and sauté the onion for 5 minutes.
2. Add the peppers and fry for 2-3 minutes more.
3. Next, add the zucchini and sauté for another 3 minutes. Remove from heat and set aside.
4. In a medium bowl beat the eggs with salt.
5. Mix the vegetables into the eggs.
6. Heat the remaining olive oil in the frying pan and pour in the egg and vegetable mixture.
7. Cook for 2-3 minutes constantly stirring.
8. Serve hot.

Servings: 4

## Cooking Times

Total Time: 25 minutes

## Nutrition Facts (per serving)

Carbs: 12,77g

Fiber: 3,26g

Protein: 12,04g

Fat: 7.94g

Calories: 165

# Electric Pressure Cooker Bok Choy Salad

### Ingredients
1 bunch bok choi, trimmed
1 cup or more water
Salt
Olive oil
Lime

### Directions
1. Place the stems in your Electric pressure cooker and pour one cup, or more water to just-cover the stems.
2. Close and lock the lid of the pressure cooker. Turn the heat up to high and when the cooker reaches pressure, lower to the heat to the minimum required by the cooker to maintain pressure.
3. Cook for 5-7 minutes at high pressure.
4. When time is up, open the cooker by Slow releasing the pressure.
5. Pull out the leaves and stems with tongs, and put on a small serving plate.
6. Dress with salt and olive oil before serving. Sprinkle some lime juice.

Servings: 3

### Cooking Times
Total Time: 10 minutes

### Nutrition Facts (per serving)
Carbs: 6,1g
Fiber: 2,8g
Protein: 4,2g
Fat: 0,56g
Calories: 36,4

# Kale, Peppers and Crumbled Feta Omelet (Slow Cooker)

### Ingredients
8 eggs, well beaten
1 cup red peppers, diced
1/4 cup green onions (finely chopped)
1/2 cup crumbled Feta
3/4 cup  kale, chopped
2 tsp.  olive oil
1/2 tsp. Italian seasoning
Salt and freshly ground pepper, to taste
sour cream cheese or cottage (optional)

### Directions
1. In a large frying pan heat oil on medium-high.  Add chopped kale and cook about 3-4 minutes.
2. Wash and chop the red peppers.  Slice the green onions and crumble the Feta. Grease the bottom of your Slow Cooker with olive oil. Add the chopped red pepper and sliced green onion to Slow Cooker with the kale.
3. In a small bowl, beat the eggs and pour over other ingredients in Slow Cooker. Stir well and add Italian seasonings. Adjust salt and pepper to taste.
4. Cook on LOW for 2 - 3 hours. Serve hot, with a dollop of sour cream if desired.

Servings: 4

### Cooking Times
Total Time: 3 hours

### Nutrition Facts (per serving)
Carbs: 4,56g
Fiber: 1,01g
Protein: 11,78g
Fat: 23,87g
Calories: 279,34

# Almond Buns

**Ingredients**

3 almond flour

5 Tbs butter, unsalted

2 eggs

1.5 tsp. sweetener of your choice (optional)

1.5 tsp. baking powder

**Directions**

1. Preheat oven to 350F.
2. Combine the dry ingredients in a bowl.
3. In a separate bowl, whisk the eggs.
4. Melt butter, add to mixture and whisk well.
5. Divide mixture equally into 6 parts and place in a greased baking dish.
6. Bake for 12-15 minutes.
7. Let cool on a wire rack.

Servings: 3

Cooking Time: 20 minutes

**Nutrition Facts (per serving)**

Carbs: 2,44g

Fiber: 0,2g

Protein: 4,45g

Fat: 22,43g

Calories: 225,58

# Mini Ham Omelets Muffins

**Ingredients**
11 oz Ham Steak
10 green onions Green Onions
12 Eggs
1/2 cup of Heavy cream
9 slices mushrooms
9 Slices Cheddar Cheese
coconut oil for greasing
Salt, Pepper, Onion Powder, Garlic Powder to taste

**Directions**
1. Preheat oven to 350F. Grease the muffin pan with coconut oil.
2. Dice the ham steak, slice the green onions and wash the mushrooms.
3. In a deep bowl, beat the eggs. Add in the heavy cream and spices along with ham cubes and sliced green onions.
4. Adjust salt, pepper and spices to taste.
5. Fill each cavity of muffin pan with the egg mixture.
6. Bake in oven for 4-5 minutes.
7. Remove from the oven and add the mushrooms on the top
8. Cook for 8-9 more minutes or until the eggs are mostly set.
9. Add Cheddar cheese and cook for 1 more minute.
10. Serve hot.

Servings: 18

**Cooking Times**
Total Time: 25 minutes

**Nutrition Facts (per serving)**
Carbs: 1,54g
Fiber: 0,32g
Protein: 11,69g
Fat: 11,1g
Calories: 153,55

# Nonpareil Bacon Waffles

**Ingredients**

4 slices bacon

2 eggs

3 cup almond flour

5 Tbsp. melted butter or ghee

1.5 tsp. baking powder

1.5 tsp. sweetener of your choice

**Directions**

1. Microwave the butter and set aside.
2. In a frying pan, cook the bacon until crisp.
3. First, mix the dry ingredients first (almond flour, baking powder and sweetener of your choice)
4. Add the two eggs and mix thoroughly. Add the melted butter and mix.
5. Preheat the waffle maker.
6. When it is preheated, open it, fill with batter and place 2 slices of bacon over top.
7. Close and flip the waffle maker, when it beeps, flip it over and remove the waffle with a fork.
8. Serve hot.

Servings: 2

**Cooking Times**

Total Time: 15 minutes

**Nutrition Facts (per serving)**

Carbs: 5,1g

Fiber: 2,65g

Protein: 8,35g

Fat: 24,97g

Calories: 323,24

# Power Greens and Sausage Casserole

## Ingredients

12 eggs
1 1/4 lbs chicken or turkey sausage
1 cup kale leaves, chopped
1 cup  arugula leaves, chopped
2 cups spinach, finely chopped
2 small zucchini - peeled
1 green onion, chopped
1/4 cup coconut milk
1/2 Tbsp. coconut oil
1 tsp. garlic powder
1 tsp. sea salt
1 tsp. pepper

## Directions

1.  Heat oven to 365 degrees. Grease casserole dish with coconut oil.
2.  In a frying pan,  melt coconut oil over medium heat, Add in sausage and stir with a wooden spoon. Cook for two to three minutes.
3.  In a big bowl beat eggs.
4.  Chop the green onion and peeled the zucchini. Mix into eggs with seasoning,  all greens and coconut milk.
5.  Pour in egg mixture and stir in sausage. Adjust the salt and pepper to taste. Cook for 45 minutes.
6.  Cover with foil and cook for 10-15 minutes more. Serve hot.

Servings: 10

## Cooking Times

Total Time: 20 minutes

## Nutrition Facts (per serving)

Carbs: 11,88g
Fiber: 1,48g
Protein: 12,19g
Fat: 7,98g
Calories: 165,48

123

# Radish, Bacon and Egg Scramble

**Ingredients**
6 oz radishes
4 oz Cheddar cheese
8 oz flank steak
2 oz bacon
4 eggs
Salt and Pepper to taste

**Directions**
1. Preheat oven to 450 degrees F. Wash the radishes, then cut the ends and quarter. Set aside.
2. In a frying pan, cook the flank steak for 5 minutes flipping from one side to another.
3. Pan fry the radishes and bacon in a cast iron skillet for about 5-6 minutes or until the radishes turn golden brown
4. Slice the flank steak and add into the pan.
5. Add the cheese and break the eggs into the mixture, season to taste and cook for one to two minutes.
6. Transfer to the oven and cook for 12 minutes until the eggs are set to the desired leve.
7. Serve and enjoy!

Servings: 4

**Cooking Times**
Total Time: 25 minutes

**Nutrition Facts (per serving)**
Carbs: 2,26g
Fiber: 0,68g
Protein: 27,42g
Fat: 22,04g
Calories: 348,58

# Sautéed Cabbage and Brussels Sprouts (Electric Pressure Cooker)

### Ingredients
4 medium beets
1-1/2 lbs cabbage, cut into wedges
1-1/2 lbs Brussels sprouts
8 large cloves garlic, left unpeeled
3 Tbsp. olive oil
1 Tbsp. chopped fresh thyme
1/2 tsp. salt, plus more to taste
1/4 tsp. freshly ground black pepper

### Directions
1. In your Electric Pressure Cooker add chopped vegetables, oil, salt and freshly ground black pepper.
2. Select SAUTE and cook under HIGH pressure for 15 minutes.
3. When ready, select natural release. Carefully open the lid.
4. Transfer all vegetables from the cooker to the serving plate, toss well and serve.

Servings: 6

### Cooking Times
Total Time: 15 minutes

### Nutrition Facts (per serving)
Total Carbs: 16,11g
Fiber: 6,57g
Protein: 6,2g
Fat: 8,31g
Calories: 160,91

# Simple Bacon Pepper Pot

**Ingredients**
6 slices bacon
4 Eggs
1 small green pepper
Jalapeno pepper, sliced
1 green onion

**Directions**
1. Slice the pepper, green onion and jalapeno into thin strips.
2. In a frying pan, cook the vegetables about 2-3 minutes until browned.
3. Chop the bacon in a food processor until it breaks into chunks.
4. Mix all the ingredients together.
5. Cook the hash until the bacon is approaching crisp.
6. Arrange on a plate and top with a fried egg!
7. Serve and enjoy!

Servings: 2
Cooking Time: 25 minutes

**Nutrition Facts (per serving)**
Carbs: 4,41g
Fiber: 1,44g
Protein: 23,33g
Fat: 29,87g
Calories: 499

# Sour and Spicy Goat Skewers

### Ingredients

1 lb boneless goat loin, cut into cubes

2 Tbsp. lime juice (freshly squeezed)

1 cup coconut yogurt

1/4 tsp. ground ginger

3/4 tsp. turmeric

1/2 tsp. ground cumin

1 Tbs ground coriander

1/2 tsp. salt

Skewers

### Directions

1. In a medium bowl, stir together coconut yogurt, lime juice and all seasonings; mix well.
2. Add the goat meat cubes to the bowl, stir to coat with the marinade, cover and refrigerate for 6-8 hours.
3. Remove the meat from the marinade, pat lightly with paper towels to dry.
4. Place meat evenly on the skewers. Grill over medium-hot coals, turning frequently, for about 10 minutes until nicely brown.
5. Serve and enjoy without guilty.

Servings: 2

### Cooking Times

Inactive Time: 10 minutes

Total Time: 25 minutes

### Nutrition Facts (per serving)

Carbs: 12,24g

Fiber: 1,25g

Protein: 26,77g

Fat: 9,79g

Calories: 342,93

# Sour Sausages with Shallots and Kalamata Olives

**Ingredients**

1 lb sausages chopped

4 shallots, finely chopped

1/2 cup lemon juice (2 lemons)

16 black and green Kalamata olives

2 Tbsp. whole grain mustard

4 Tbsp. extra virgin olive oil

salt and ground black pepper to taste

**Directions**

1. Preheat oven to 400F. Grease an roasting pan and place in the sausages and chopped shallots.
2. Roast for 20 minutest.
3. When ready, remove the meat from the sausages and season with salt and freshly ground pepper to taste
4. Pour the lemon juice into the roasting tin.
5. Add in the mustard and chopped olives and simmer gently for 2-3 minutes. Pour lemon mixture over the sausages and shallots.
6. Place on serving plate and serve.

Servings: 6

**Cooking Times**

Total Time: 30 minutes

**Nutrition Facts (per serving)**

Carbs: 14,9g

Fiber: 0,42g

Protein: 18,48

Fat: 16,67g

Calories: 408

# Spinach and Cheese Stuffed Mushrooms

**Ingredients**

12 large mushroom caps with stems

1 cream cheese

1 cup cooked, chopped spinach

1 Tbsp. garlic, minced

1 tsp. red pepper flakes

2 scallions, finely chopped

1 tsp. salt

1 tsp. fresh cracked pepper

3 tsp. extra virgin olive oil

2 Tbsp. almond, ground

2 Tbsp. Parmesan cheese

1 tsp. granulated garlic

1 Tbsp. fresh flat leaf parsley, finely chopped

**Directions**

1. Preheat the oven to 400 degrees F.
2. First, remove the mushrooms stems. Chop the stems finely.
3. Heat a frying skillet with 2 teaspoons of olive oil and cook the mushrooms stems for 5 minutes.
4. In a bowl, combine the cream cheese, red pepper flakes, scallions, chopped spinach, minced garlic, cooked mushroom stems, salt & pepper. In a small bowl, combine ground almonds, parmesan cheese, parsley and granulated garlic.
5. Fill the mushroom cavities with cheese and mushrooms mixture. Sprinkle the ground almonds mixture over each mushroom.
6. Drizzle the remaining 1 teaspoon of oil over the filling in the mushroom caps. Bake in oven about 12 minutes. Serve hot.

Servings: 6

**Cooking Times**

Cooking Time: 12 minutes

Total Time: 20 minutes

**Nutrition Facts (per serving)**

Carbs: 11,36g

Fiber: 5,24g

Protein: 11,75g

Fat: 6,36g

Calories: 138,32

# Spinach-Chard Puree with Almonds

**Ingredients**

1 lb baby spinach leaves

1/2 lb Swiss chard, tough stems removed, tender stems and leaves torn into 2" pieces

1 cup cauliflower flowerets (1 cup)

1 leek

1/4 cup  extra virgin olive oil

3 cups water

4 Tbsp. toasted almond slivers

1/4 cup tofu cheese, cubed

salt and black ground pepper to taste

**Directions**

1.  Wash the leek and cut it into thick slices.
2.  Heat the olive oil in a saucepan and cook the leek and cauliflower for about 2-3 minutes.
3.  Add the chard and cleaned spinach leaves, water and a pinch of salt and pepper to taste. Bring to the boil and let it simmer for 15 minutes.
4.  Remove from the heat and place the vegetables in a food processor. Blend into a very smooth soup.
5.  Pour the mixture into bowls, place some tofu cubes on top and generously sprinkle with ground toasted almonds.

Servings: 10

**Cooking Times**

Total Time: 35 minutes

**Nutrition Facts (per serving)**

Carbs: 6,92g

Fiber: 1,88g

Protein: 5,24g

Fat: 1,69g

Calories: 47,47

130

# Lunch Recipes

# Baked Creamy Cauliflower-Broccoli Chicken

**Ingredients**

2 boneless chicken breasts
1 cup chicken broth
3 cups cauliflower
3 cups broccoli, steamed and chopped
2 cups shredded Cheddar cheese
1 cup heavy cream
1 small yellow onion
1/2 Tbsp. minced garlic
1 tsp. lemon juice
1/2 cup mayonnaise
3 Tbsp. ghee
fresh parsley, chopped
salt and fresh pepper to taste

**Directions**

1. Preheat the oven to 350 degrees.
2. In a deep saucepot boil chicken breast until the chicken is cooked through.
3. Meanwhile, in a frying pan with the ghee cook up the garlic and onions on a low heat. Add all spices one by one stirring frequently.
4. While that's cooking, in a food processor blend up your cauliflower.
5. When the onions are soft, add the cauliflower. Cook for 2-3 minutes. Add in the chicken broth. Cook, covered for about 10 minutes.
6. Add the heavy cream and lemon juice and let simmer uncovered on low for about 10 minutes more. At the end, add in mayonnaise and stir.
7. Pull apart your chicken and add half of chicken into the cauliflower cream mixture.
8. Use the other half to line the bottom of an 8x8 casserole dish. On top of the chicken, layer in chopped broccoli.
9. Top with the cauliflower cream mixture.
10. Cover it with cheddar cheese.

11. Bake in preheated oven for 40 minutes. Serve hot.

Servings: 8
Cooking Times: 1 hour and 15 minutes

**Nutrition Facts (per serving)**
Calories 365
Fat 29,17g
Carbs 9,25g
Fiber 0,95g
Protein 17,9g

# Baked Manchego Chicken Wings

### Ingredients
20 frozen wings
1 cup of grated Manchego cheese (or Parmesan, Asagio...)
2 Tbsp. Olive oil
2 tsp. dried oregano
1/2 Tbsp. garlic powder
1 tsp. garlic salt

### Directions
1. Preheat oven to 450F.
2. In a baking pan greased with olive oil place frozen chicken wings. Sprinkle with salt and oregano.
3. Bake for 35 minutes.
4. Remove from oven and toss in a bowl with another tbsp. of garlic oil until coated.
5. Sprinkle with grated Manchego cheese and garlic powder.
6. Serve hot.

Servings: 4

Cooking Times
Total Time: 45 minutes

### Nutrition Facts (per serving)
Calories 446
Fat 33,51g
Carbs 2,67g
Fiber 0,68g
Protein 32,34g

# Baked Pork Chops in Sweet-Sour Marinade

**Ingredients**
4.48 lbs. pork chops
1 cup Apple cider vinegar
1 cup Erythritol
4 Tbsp. soy Sauce
1 cup Apple Cider Vinegar
1 tsp. ginger
1 tsp. pepper
coconut or olive oil for greasing

**Directions**
1.  Preheat oven to 350F.
2.  In a food processor, add all of the ingredients (except the pork chops).
3.  Blend well to make the marinade.
4.  In a greased pan place all of the pork chops and pour the marinade over it.
5.  Cook for 60 minutes in a preheated oven flipping after 30 minutes.
6.  Once ready place chops on a serving plate and enjoy your lunch!

Servings: 10

**Cooking Times**
Preparation Time: 10 minutes
Total Time: 1 hour and 10 minutes

**Nutrition Facts (per serving)**
Calories 307
Fat 6,97g
Carbs 11,43g
Fiber 0,08g
Protein 45,89g

# Bolognese Squash Spaghetti

## Ingredients
1 lb. ground beef
2 1/2 cups Spaghetti squash
1 egg
3/4 cup Marinara Sauce
1 cup grated Parmesan cheese
1 cups shredded mozzarella cheese
1 tsp. chili powder
1/2 tsp. oregano
1/2 tsp. parsley (fresh and chopped)
1/2 tsp. basil
1 tsp. crushed red pepper flakes
2 tsp. of garlic minced
sea salt and ground fresh pepper to taste
ghee

## Directions
1.  Preheat oven to 350F.
2.  Roast your spaghetti squash in the oven for about one hour.
3.  In a saucepan, heat Marinara sauce; add oregano, parsley, basil and red pepper flakes. Cover and let simmer for a few minutes. Mix meatball ingredients in a bowl and roll into quarter-sized mini meatballs.
4.  In a frying pan heat the ghee and cook meatballs covered. After 3 minutes, flip when halfway browned.
5.  Once the meatballs are cooked through, transfer them into the sauce. In a small bread pan, layer spaghetti squash, sauce, meatballs and mozzarella. Bake on 25 for 30 minutes. Serve hot.

Servings: 5
Cooking Time: 45 minutes

## Nutrition Facts (per serving)
Calories 446
Fat 30,63g
Carbs 9,1g
Fiber 0,93g
Protein 32,33g

# Cheesy Zoodles with Fresh Basil

**Ingredients**

2 cups zucchini noodles (zoodles)

2 Tbsp. fresh chopped basil

1/4 cup Pecorino Romano cheese, shaved

1/4 cup Grana Padano cheese, grated

3 Tbsp. salted butter

3 cloves mashed garlic

1 tsp. red pepper flakes

1 Tbsp. chopped red pepper

1 Tbsp. coconut oil

Salt and fresh cracked pepper to taste

**Directions**

1. In a frying pan over medium heat, melt butter and coconut oil. Add in garlic, chopped red pepper and red pepper flakes. Sauté for 1 minute only.
2. Add in the zoodles and let cook for 1-2 minutes. Turn off heat and toss with fresh basil. Toss slightly.
3. Add in Pecorino Romano cheese and toss.
4. Finally, sprinkle on top with grated Grana Padano cheese.
5. Serve immediately.

Servings: 3

**Cooking Times**

Total Time: 15 minutes

**Nutrition Facts (per serving)**

Calories 314

Fat 26,38g

Carbs 6,18g

Fiber 2,3g

Protein 15,78g

# Spicy Spinach Casserole

## Ingredients
2 1/2 cups spinach, drained
2 lbs. ground pork/beef
16 oz. cream cheese
10 Tbsp. sour cream
8 oz. Emmenthal Cheese, shredded
2 cups pepper sauce
1 onion
1 red pepper
4 tsp. Taco seasoning
Sliced Jalapeños to taste

## Directions
1. Preheat oven to 350F. Grease one 8" square & a 9x13 baking dish.
2. Chop and sauté some jalapenos with chopped peppers and onions. Transfer to a bowl and set aside.
3. Add the spinach to the pan and cook until thawed completely. Move the spinach to the prep bowl
4. In a frying pan, add ground pork/meat and cook until browned well. Add taco seasoning and mix. Remove from fire and set aside.
5. In a bowl, add sour cream, mozzarella and cream cheese. Add in peppers, onion, spinach and ground meat.
6. Transfer this mix to prepared and greased baking dish and bake for 40 minutes. Serve hot or cold.

Servings: 10

## Cooking Times
Cooking Time: 45 minutes
Total Time: 1 hour

## Nutrition Facts (per serving)
Calories 460
Fat 37,26g
Carbs 5,33g
Fiber 0,84g
Protein 25,63g

# Cabbage with Ground Beef Stew

**Ingredients**
1 1/2 lb. ground beef
2 lbs. green cabbage
1/2 cup unsalted butter
1/2 cup water
3 cups pasta sauce
Salt and pepper to taste

**Directions**
1. In a food processor, shred quartered cabbage.
2. In a saucepan, melt the butter and add the cabbage, water and salt and pepper to taste.
3. Cover and cook for 12-15 minutes, stirring occasionally
4. In a meanwhile, in a frying pan brown the ground beefs.
5. Once browned, add the beef to the cabbage and stir well. Finally, add the pasta sauce and stir. Serve hot.

Servings: 10

**Cooking Times**
Cooking Time: 15 minutes
Total Time: 25 minutes

**Nutrition Facts (per serving)**
Calories 307
Fat 22,29g
Total Carbs 12,34g
Fiber 3,6g
Protein 14,9g

# Three Cheeses & Beef Pizza

**Ingredients**

1 lb. ground beef

2 beef sausage

1 cup chopped Romaine lettuce

2 Tbsp. yellow onions

3 Tbsp. chopped dill pickle

1 1/2 cups Parmesan cheese

1/2 cup Colby cheese, shredded

1 1/2 cups Cheddar, shredded

1/4 Tbsp. paprika

1/4 tsp. Old Bay seasoning

1/4 tsp. garlic powder

1/4 tsp. onion powder

2 Tbsp. organic Thousand island dressing

mustard to taste

1/4 tsp. sea salt

1/4 tsp. ground black pepper

olive oil

2 Tbsp. water

**Directions**

1. In a frying pan greased with olive oil, add 1 cup Parmesan cheese evenly and then on top, 1 cup shredded Cheddar.
2. Leave to cook 2-3 minutes; use a spatula to lift the edges and underneath of the pizza, and slide out onto a flat surface. Allow to cool.
3. Repeat the same process, for the second pizza crust. Once done, set both cheese crusts aside.
4. Use a spatula and evenly spread Thousand Island dressing over the cheese crusts
5. In a frying pan add ground beef and cook until browned. Add old bay seasoning, garlic powder, onion powder paprika, 2 tbsp. water, salt, ground black pepper to taste. Mix and set to simmer on low.
6. Finally, add in chopped hot dogs into slices and simmer for about 4-5 minutes.
7. Place chopped lettuce over your pizza crust.

8. In a bowl, place your pickles, onions, Colby cheese, and set aside.
9. On top of each cheese crust, add about a cup of the ground meat and hotdog mixture and spread evenly .Sprinkle with onions and pickles.
10. Drizzle mustard on top.
11. Sprinkle with more cheese if you like and serve.

Servings: 7
Cooking Time: 20 minutes

**Nutrition Facts (per serving)**
Calories 511
Fat 39,9g
Carbs 2,78g
Fiber 0,42g
Protein 33,59g

# Chicken Angel Eggs

**Ingredients**
1 cup chicken, finely chopped
6 eggs
3 Tbsp. mayonnaise
1 Tbsp. chopped onion
1/2 tsp. dill
1/2 tsp. parsley
1 tsp. Dijon mustard
1/2 tsp. pepper mix seasoning
old bay seasoning
salt and black ground pepper to taste

**Directions**
1. In a bowl, mix all rest of ingredients (except eggs) until well mixed. Refrigerate the chicken salad for 10-15 minutes.
2. Boil your eggs. Shell, cool, and cut in half. Save or toss your yolks.
3. Fill your egg halves with chicken salad. Sprinkle with Old Bay or some other seasoning of your taste. Serve.

Servings: 4

Cooking Times
Total Time: 25 minutes

**Nutrition Facts (per serving)**
Calories 161
Fat 11,22g
Carbs 3,73g
Fiber 0,08g
Protein 10,82g

# Monterey Jack Steak

**Ingredients**

1 lb. shaved steak

4 slices Monterey Jack cheese

2 Tbsp. mayonnaise

1 Tbsp. Dijon mustard

1/4 cup chopped green peppers

1/4 cup chopped onions

1 Tbsp. minced garlic

1 Tbsp. olive oil

1 Tbsp. ghee

**Directions**

1. In a large frying pan add ghee and olive oil to warm over medium heat. Add onions, green peppers and garlic. Cook until soft, about 2-3 minutes. Add shaved steak and cook until browned several minutes.
2. Turn heat down to low. Add Dijon mustard and mayonnaise and mix.
3. Add Monterey Jack cheese on top of the steak and let melt until cheese is melted throughout, about 1 minute.
4. Serve hot.

Servings: 4

**Cooking Times**

Total Time: 20 minutes

**Nutrition Facts (per serving)**

Calories 345

Fat 25,2g

Carbs 4,35g

Fiber 0,48g

Protein 24,51g

# Pumpkin Chili

### Ingredients
2 lbs. ground beef
1 can (15 oz.) pumpkin puree
1 Tbsp. pumpkin pie spice
3 cups 100% tomato juice
3 tomatoes, diced
1 red bell pepper
1 yellow onion
2 tsp. cumin
1 Tbsp. chili powder
2 tsp. cayenne pepper
ghee or coconut oil

### Directions
1. In a large frying pan greased with ghee or coconut oil, brown the meat over medium heat.
2. Chop the onion and pepper and add into the pot with the meat. Cook 3-5 minutes or until the onions become translucent.
3. Add in the rest of the ingredients and let simmer on LOW for 30 minutes.
4. Season chili with salt and pepper to taste and cook for another 30 minutes.
5. Serve hot.

Servings: 8

### Cooking Times
Total Time: 1 hour and 20 minutes

### Nutrition Facts (per serving)
Calories 354
Fat 25,24g
Carbs 9,87g
Fiber 2,14g 9%
Protein 21,87g 44%

# Slow Cooker Roast and Chicken Stew

**Ingredients**

3 lb. pot roast

1 lb. chicken breast (boiled and shredded)

6 oz. Italian sweet sausage

2 cups beef broth

1 cup chicken stock

1/2 medium onion (chopped)

1 can (11 oz.) low carb diced tomatoes

1/4 tsp. thyme

1/4 tsp. celery salt

1 Tbsp. coconut oil

1 tsp. basil

2 tsp. dried dill weed

2 tsp. garlic powder

2 tsp. pepper

1 Tbsp. garlic salt

1 tsp. minced garlic

1 Tbsp. oregano

1 Tbsp. powdered buttermilk

4 tsp. onion powder

4 tsp. dried parsley

5 tsp. red pepper flakes

2 tsp. hot sauce

**Directions**

1. At the bottom of your Slow Cooker place roast, chicken breast and Italian sausages. Add on the top all other ingredients and stir lightly.
2. Close the lid and cook on LOW for about 6-8 hours.
3. Once ready, flavor to taste with some additional hot sauce, salt and pepper to your own liking and serve hot.

Servings: 10

**Nutrition Facts (per serving)**

Calories 467

Fat 36,21g

Carbs 3,76g

Fiber 1,03g

Protein 30,11g

# Mediterranean Pecorino Romano Breaded Cutlets

### Ingredients
6 pork cutlets
1/2 cup grated Pecorino Romano cheese
2 Tbsp. fresh lemon juice
2 Tbsp. water
1 Tbsp. olive oil
1 Tbsp. green pepper, minced
1 Tbsp. garlic, minced
salt and ground black pepper to taste

### Directions
1. Heat a greasing frying pan to medium.
2. In a bowl pour water, lemon juice, olive oil, minced pepper and garlic. Season the salt and pepper to taste. Mix well.
3. In a separate bowl pour grated Pecorino Romano cheese.
4. Dip each cutlet first in liquid dressing and then in cheese.
5. Cook cutlets in pan for about 15-20 minutes. Serve hot.

Servings: 3

Cooking Times
Total Time: 30 minutes

### Nutrition Facts (per serving)
Calories 395
Fat 38,78g
Carbs 2,5g
Fiber 0,16g
Protein 9,1g

# Oriental Garlicky Chicken Thighs

**Ingredients**

4 chicken thighs
16 whole cloves of garlic
2 Tbsp. ghee
2 Tbsp. juice of one fresh lemon
1 cup of baby carrots
1 onion, cut into quarters
2 tomatoes cut in half
3 Tbsp. garlic olive oil (or extra-virgin olive oil)
oregano
Salt and pepper

**Directions**

1. Preheat oven to 500F degrees.
2. Grease the bottom of a non-stick frying pan with garlic olive oil (or olive oil). Add in the chicken thighs together.
3. In between the thighs, wedge in the garlic gloves, onions, tomatoes and baby carrots.
4. Pour the lemon juice over the chicken thighs. Drizzle ghee and garlic oil over the thighs.
5. Sprinkle oregano over the dish and season with salt and pepper to taste.
6. Bake in preheated oven for 25-30 minutes.
7. Reduce heat to 350 and cook for 20 minutes more.
8. Once ready, let cool for 5 minutes on a wire rack and serve hot.

Servings: 4

**Cooking Times**
Total Time: 1 hour and 5 minutes

**Nutrition Facts (per serving)**
Calories 237
Fat 14,52g
Carbs 8,97g
Fiber 1,31g
Protein 17,68g

# Pordenone Cauliflower Lasagna

**Ingredients**

12 chicken thighs

30 oz. chopped cauliflower

6 green onions

1 onion, chopped

1 green pepper

6 bacon Slices

1 cup Cream Cheese

1/2 cup heavy cream

8 oz. Pepper Jack Cheese, shredded

8 oz. Cheddar Cheese, shredded

1 Tbsp. garlic, minced

salt and pepper to taste

**Directions**

1. Preheat oven to350F.
2. Chop up a head of cauliflower into florets. Cook the cauliflower in the microwave on the vegetable setting. Set aside.
3. In a pan on stovetop, toss the chicken thighs with salt and pepper to taste. Add some water to about mid-thigh and cook for 60 minutes. Chop up the onions and peppers and pan fry it.
4. Add all of the other ingredients, reserving 2 oz. Cheddar and 2 oz. of Pepper Jack Cheese.
5. Add the mixture into a large, greased casserole dish and top with the remaining cheese.
6. Cover with foil and cook for 30 minutes. Serve hot.

Servings: 10

**Cooking Times**

Preparation Time: 20 minutes

Cooking Time: 1 hour and 30 minutes

**Nutrition Facts (per serving)**

Calories 486

Fat 35,69g

Carbs 13,73g

Fiber 2,2g

Protein 28,09g

# Roasted Chicken & Prosciutto with Brussels sprouts

**Ingredients**

2 lbs. chicken tenderloins

4 oz. prosciutto

12 oz. Brussels sprouts

1/2 cup chicken broth

1 1/2 cups heavy cream

1 tsp. minced garlic

1 lemon, quartered and seeded

ghee or coconut oil for frying

**Directions**

1. Preheat oven to 400 degrees.
2. Cut the Brussels sprouts in half and boil for 5 minutes. Remove from heat and set aside.
3. In a frying pan add 1/2 cup chicken broth and bring to a boil on medium. After that, add heavy cream, minced garlic and lemon and let simmer for 5-10 minutes stirring frequently. Remove from heat and set aside.
4. In a separate frying pan, heat up some ghee and add chicken. Cook on medium high heat for several minutes, and then add chopped prosciutto until chicken is cooked.
5. In a small casserole dish (9×9) and layer from bottom to top: Brussels sprouts, chicken, prosciutto, lemon cream sauce on top.
6. Bake in preheated oven for 20 minutes. Serve hot.

Servings: 6

**Cooking Times**

Total Time: 40 minutes

**Nutrition Facts (per serving)**

Calories 333

Fat 16,76g

Carbs 5,2g

Fiber 1,48g

Protein 39,47g

# Roquefort Spinach, Zoodles and Bacon Salad

### Ingredients
4 cups of zucchini noodles
1 cup fresh broccoli
1/2 cup crumbled bacon
1 cup fresh spinach
1/3 cup Roquefort, bleu cheese, crumbled
1/3 cup bleu cheese dressing
fresh cracked pepper (to taste)

### Directions
1. In a deep bowl add all the ingredients together and toss slightly with wooden spoon.
2. Serve and enjoy!

Servings: 5
Cooking Time: 5 minutes

### Nutrition Facts (per serving)
Calories 81,
Fat 3,15g
Carbs 9,58g
Fiber 3,05g
Protein 6,07g

# Sour Avocado and Chicken Moussaka

**Ingredients**

8 chicken thighs, cooked

1 cup sour cream

1 cup Parmesan Cheese

4 avocados

1 onion

1 green pepper

1 Tbsp. cayenne peppers sauce

salt and ground pepper to taste

coconut oil for greasing

**Directions**

1. Preheat oven to 350 F. Grease a baking dish with coconut oil.
2. In a pot cook your chicken thighs about 35 minutes. Peel avocados, cut in half, and slice into thin strips.
3. Line the bottom with avocado slices. In a small pan fry chopped peppers and onions until caramelized.
4. Add the chicken into a large bowl and chop it. Add remaining ingredients and mix well.
5. Spoon mixture over the avocado slices. Bake for 20 minutes.
6. Serve hot.

Servings: 8

**Cooking Times**

Total Time: 35 minutes

**Nutrition Facts (per serving)**

Calories 345

Fat 25,32g

Carbs 11,08g

Fiber 6,45g

Protein 20,98g

# Spicy Italian Sausage and Spinach Casserole

**Ingredients**
16 oz. spicy Italian sausage
2 1/2 cups frozen spinach
12 eggs
8 oz. Cheddar
1 onion
9 oz. Cherry Tomatoes
1 green pepper, chopped
12 Tbsp. Heavy Cream
Garlic powder
Onion Powder
Salt and ground pepper to taste
coconut or olive oil

**Directions**
1. Preheat oven to 350F. Grease casserole dish with coconut or olive oil.
2. In microwave cook the spinach. Chop the spicy Italian sausage and cook in a frying pan until browned. Remove to the big bowl and set aside.
3. In the same frying pan, cook the sliced onion and pepper. Transfer to the bowl with spinach.
4. Whisk together the eggs, spices and a heavy cream. Add the cheese to the bowl and combine, then add the egg mixture and combine.
5. Transfer to a greased casserole dish and add cherry tomatoes.
6. Cook in preheated oven for 50 minutes. Serve hot.

Servings: 10
**Cooking Times**: 1 hour and 5 minutes

**Nutrition Facts (per serving)**
Calories 343
Fat 25,91g
Carbs 6,27g
Fiber 2,5g
Protein 22,68g

# Squash Spaghetti Lasagna Dish

**Ingredients**

2 1/2 lbs. ground beef

2 large Spaghetti Squash

7 ounces whole milk Ricotta Cheese

7 ounces Mozzarella cheese, sliced

4 cups Marinara sauce

coconut or olive oil for greasing

**Directions**

1. Preheat oven to 375F. Grease a large baking dish with coconut or olive oil.
2. Split the Spaghetti Squash and lay face down into large glass dish and fill with water. Bake for 40-45 minutes.
3. While the Spaghetti Squash is cooking, in a large saucepan cook the ground meat and the marinara sauce. Once combined, set aside.
4. When the Spaghetti Squash is done scrap the meat of the squash to from spaghetti.
5. Assembly the lasagna in a large greased pan, start with a layer of Spaghetti Squash, then the meat sauce, then slices of mozzarella, then ricotta, then repeats until ingredients are exhausted.
6. Bake for 30-35 35 minutes until the top layer of cheese is browning. Serve hot or keep refrigerated.

Servings: 14

Cooking Times

Total Time: 1 hour and 30 minutes

**Nutrition Facts (per serving)**

Calories 437,

Fat 27,77g

Carbs 16,49g

Fiber 1,91g

Protein 28,79g

# Tuna Avocado Bites

### Ingredients
Mayonnaise (1/4 cup)
Parmesan cheese (1/4 cup)
Garlic powder (1/2 teaspoon)
Salt
Canned Tuna (10 oz., drained)
Avocado (1, cubed)
Almond flour (1/3 cup)
Onion powder (1/4 teaspoon)
Coconut oil (1/2 cup)

### Directions
1. Combine all ingredients in a bowl except oil and avocado.
2. Add avocado and fold, use hands to form balls and dust with flour.
3. Heat oil in a pot and fry tuna bites until golden all over.
4. Serve.

Servings: 12

### Nutrition Facts (per serving)
Calories 135
Fats 11.8g
Protein 6.2 g
Fiber 1.2g

**Note:** 3-4 bites would be good for a serving. Paired with a salad and lunch is complete.

# Crispy Baked Tofu and Bok Choy Salad

**Ingredients**

*For Tofu:*
Soy sauce (1 tablespoon)
Water (1 tablespoon)
Rice wine vinegar (1 tablespoon)
Tofu (15 oz., extra firm)
Sesame oil (1 tablespoon)
Garlic (2 teaspoons)
Lemon juice (from ½ lemon)

*For Salad:*
Green onion (1 stalk)
Coconut oil (3 tablespoons)
Sambal Olek (1 tablespoon)
Lime juice (from ½ lime)
Bok Choy (9 oz.)
Cilantro (2 tablespoons, chopped)
Soy sauce (2 tablespoons)
Peanut butter (1 tablespoon)
Stevia liquid (7 drops)

**Directions**
1. Wrap tofu in a clean cloth and press for 6 hours until dry.
2. Combine soy sauce, water, vinegar, lemon juice, sesame oil and garlic in a bowl and cube tofu. Add to marinade, cover with plastic and put aside for 30 minutes or overnight if possible.
3. Set oven to 350 °F. Use parchment paper to line a baking sheet and place marinated tofu on sheet. Bake for 35 minutes.
4. Prepare dressing for salad by combining all ingredients except bok choy. Chop bok choy finely and toss in dressing.
5. Top bok choy with baked tofu and serve.

Servings: 3
**Nutrition Facts (per serving)**
Calories 442
Net Carbs 5.7g
Fats 35g
Protein 25 g
Fiber 1.7g

# Homemade Meatballs

### Ingredients
500g ground beef
1 whole egg
Almond flour (1/2 cups)
2 cloves of garlic, minced
Oregano, dried (1 teaspoon)
Thyme, dried (1 teaspoon)
1 cup mozzarella cheese, shredded
Salt and pepper to taste
Homemade marinara sauce (1/2 cups)

### Directions
1. Preheat oven at 450F.
2. In a large bowl, place the ground beef, egg, almond flour, garlic, oregano, thyme, and season with salt and pepper. Also add the cheese.
3. Using your hands, mix all the ingredients together; making sure that everything is well combined.
4. Create 25 pcs of meat balls and lay them on a baking sheet lined with parchment paper.
5. Cook in the oven to cook for 15 minutes or until golden brown.
6. Serve the meatballs with marinara sauce.

Servings: 12

### Nutrition Facts (per serving)
Calories: 117
Net Carbs: 0.9
Fat: 9.3g
Protein: 7g

# BBQ Chicken Soup

**Ingredients**

*For Soup Base:*
Chicken thighs (3)
Salt
Chicken broth (1 ½ cups)
Chili seasoning (2 teaspoons)
Olive oil (2 tablespoons)
Beef broth (1 ½ cups)
Black pepper

*For BBQ Sauce:*
Ketchup (1/4 cup, reduced sugar)
Dijon mustard (2 tablespoons)
Hot sauce (1 tablespoon)
Worcestershire sauce (1 teaspoon)
Onion powder (1 teaspoon)
Red chili flakes (1 teaspoon)
Butter (1/4 cup)
Tomato paste (1/4 cup)
Soy sauce (1 tablespoon)
Liquid smoke (2 ½ teaspoons)
Garlic powder (1 ½ teaspoons)
Chili powder (1 teaspoon)
Cumin (1 teaspoon)

**Directions**

1. Set oven to 400 F. Remove bones from chicken and put bones aside. Season chicken with chili seasoning and place into oven for 50 minutes.
2. Heat oil in a deep pot and add bones. Cook for 5 minutes then add beef and chicken broth; season with pepper and salt.
3. Take chicken from oven and remove skin. Add the fat to the soup and mix together. Combine BBQ sauce ingredients and add to pot. Cook for 30 minutes.
4. Combine fats in soup by using an immersion blender then shred chicken and add to soup. Cook for 20 minutes.
5. Serve topped with chicken skin. May add cheese or bell peppers.

Servings: 4

**Nutrition Facts (per serving)**
Calories 487
Net Carbs 4.3g
Fats 38.3g
Protein 24.5 g
Fiber 1.3g

# Salmon Salad in Avo Cups

**Ingredients**
1 medium-sized salmon fillet
1 pc. shallot, diced
Mayo (1/4 cups)
½ juice of lime
Fresh dill, chopped (2 tablespoons)
Ghee (1 tablespoon)
1 large avocado, sliced in half and pitted
salt and pepper to taste

**Directions**
1. Preheat oven at 400F
2. Place the salmon fillet on a baking sheet and drizzle it with ghee and juice of lime. Season with salt and pepper and place in the oven to cook for 20-25 minutes.
3. When done, allow the salmon to cook for a few minutes and shred using a fork.
4. Place the salmon in a bowl, add the diced shallot, and mix well.
5. Add the dill and mayo to the salmon mixture and combine well. Set aside.
6. Remove the insides of the avocado halves making sure that the skin is still intact to make cups.
7. Mash the avocado meat in a bowl and then add to the salmon mixture. Combine well.
8. Transfer the avocado and salmon salad back to the avocado cups and serve.

Servings: 2

**Nutrition Facts (per serving)**
Calories: 463
Net Carbs: 6.4g
Fat: 35g
Protein: 27g

# Bacon Chicken Patties

### Ingredients
Chicken breast (12 oz. can)
Bell peppers (2, medium)
Parmesan cheese (1/4 cup)
Coconut flour (3 tablespoons)
Bacon (4 slices)
Sundried Tomato pesto (1/4 cup)
Egg (1)

### Directions
1. Cook bacon until crisp, put aside until needed.
2. Put bell pepper into a processor and pulse until fine, put into a bowl and squeeze out excess liquid.
3. Put bacon and chicken into processor and pulse until thoroughly combined, transfer mixture to bowl with peppers.
4. Add egg, pesto parmesan and flour to mixture and combine.
5. Heat oil in a skillet and form patties. Add to pan and cook until golden all over.
6. Serve.

Servings: 10

### Nutrition Facts (per serving)
Calories 159
Net Carbs 1.7g
Fats 11.5g
Protein 9.9 g
Fiber 14g

# Savory Mince

**Ingredients**

Coconut oil (4 tablespoons)

1Kg Beef/Chicken/Lamb/Pork/Ostrich mince

2 Onion finely diced

Vegetables (green/red/yellow/orange peppers, mushroom, tomatoes, celery, baby marrows, spinach) finely diced (4 cups)

4 Carrots finely grated

1 Packet gluten free gravy

Tomato paste (1/2 cups)

250ml chicken stock

**Directions**

1. Heat coconut oil in a pan and fry chopped onion,
2. Add beef mince with and tomato paste and fry.
3. Add chopped vegetables and grated carrot to the cooked mince.
4. Continue to cook on a low heat until the vegetables are well cooked.
5. If your mixture seems to be drying out, keep adding chicken stock to keep at the right consistency.
6. The longer you cook this mixture, the more the flavours will infuse through the mince.
7. Add gluten free gravy

# Cheesy Bacon Spinach Log

**Ingredients**

Cheddar cheese (2 ½ cups, shredded)
Chipotle seasoning (2 tablespoons)
Bacon (30 slices)
Mrs. Dash seasoning (2 teaspoons)
Spinach (5 cups)

**Directions**

1.  Set oven to 375 °F.
2.  Place bacon in a weaving pattern on a baking sheet lined with foil and season with spices.
3.  Top bacon with cheese leaving a 1 inch space all around the edge. Add spinach and push it down and roll the bacon together into a log.
4.  Sprinkle with salt and place into oven for 60 minutes.
5.  Cool for 15 minutes and slice.
6.  Serve.

Servings: 5

**Nutrition Facts (per serving)**

Calories 432
Net Carbs 3g
Fats 38.2g
Protein 32.8 g
Fiber 3g

# Beef Sausage, Bacon & Broccoli Casserole

**Ingredients**
500 g beef sausage
1/2 head of broccoli
8 slices of bacon
Cream (1/2 cups)
Dijon mustard (1 tablespoon)
100 g grated cheddar cheese

**Directions**
1. Preheat oven to 350F
2. Slice the sausage and place in a small baking dish.
3. Slice the bacon and add to the sausage.
4. Break the broccoli into florets and arrange between the meat.
5. Mix the cream and mustard in a bowl and pour it all over the casserole, then top with the cheese.
6. Bake in the oven for 35 minutes.

Servings: 2

**Nutrition Facts (per serving)**
Calories: 300
Net Carbs: 3g
Fat: 25g
Protein: 20g

# Grilled Cheese and Ham Sandwich

## Ingredients

*For buns:*
Eggs (2)
Salted butter (1 ½ tablespoons)
Coconut flour (1 teaspoon)
Almond flour (3/4 cup)
Coconut oil (2 tablespoons)
Baking powder (1 teaspoon)
Salt (1/4 teaspoon)

*Filling:*
Deli Ham (4 slices)
Cheddar cheese (2 slices)
Butter (1 tablespoon, salted)
Muenster cheese (2 slices)

## Directions
1. Set oven to 350 °F.
2. Place almond flour, baking powder in a bowl and mix together.
3. Put coconut oil and butter in a microwavable dish and heat until melted then add to dry mix. Combine until mixture gets doughy.
4. Beat eggs and add to dough mixture then put in coconut flour.
5. Grease cupcake molds and add batter to each about ¾ ways filled. Baked for 18 minutes and take from oven, allow to cool and slice into two horizontally.
6. Use cheese and ham to fill buns, melt butter in a skillet and place sandwiches into pan. Cook for 3 minutes on each side until golden and cheese melts. Serve.

Servings: 1

## Nutrition Facts (per serving)
Calories 272
Fats 24.2g
Protein 11.3g
Fiber 3.8g

# Creamed Spinach

## Ingredients
Spinach (2 cups)
½ small onion, chopped
Water (1/4 cups)
1/2 stock cube
1 clove of garlic, chopped
Heavy cream (1/4 cups)
Butter (2 tablespoons)
Salt and pepper to taste

## Directions
1.  Place spinach and onion to a pan with water and heat over medium-high fire.
2.  Add stock cube and garlic and allow to steam for 8-10 minutes or until all the water has evaporated and the spinach is very soft.
3.  Pour in the heavy cream and butter and then season with salt and pepper. Cooking until it thickens.
4.  Using a hand-held blender blitz the spinach until fairly smooth.
5.  Serve while hot

Servings: 1

## Nutrition Facts (per serving)
Calories: 200
Net Carbs: 3g
Fat: 23g
Protein: 7g

# Cheesy Pizza

**Ingredients**
Ground beef (1/2 lb.)
Eggs (2)
Garlic powder (1 teaspoon)
Basil (1/4 teaspoon)
Turmeric (1/4 teaspoon)
Cream cheese (8 oz., room temp.)
Chorizo sausage (1)
Parmesan cheese (1/4 cup, grated)
Cumin (1/2 teaspoon)
Italian seasoning (1/2 teaspoon)
Tomato sauce (3/4 cup, low carb)
Salt & Black pepper

**Directions**
1. Set oven to 375 °F.
2. Put cream cheese, eggs, garlic powder, parmesan cheese and black pepper in a bowl and use mixer to blend until smooth.
3. Grease a baking pan and pour in cheese mixture and spread evenly; bake for 15 minutes.
4. Put beef into a skillet and cook for 5 minutes then add Italian seasoning, basil, salt, black pepper, cumin and turmeric. Cook for 10 minutes or until thoroughly cooked.
5. Take crust from oven and cool for 10 minutes then top with tomato sauce and cheese. Return to oven and bake for 10 minutes until cheese melts then top with beef.
6. Broil for an additional 5 minutes. Take from oven and cool for 10 minutes. Slice and serve.

Servings: 12 small slices

**Nutrition Facts (per serving)**
Calories 145
Net Carbs 1.2g
Fats 11.3g
Protein 8.2 g
Fiber 3g

# Hearty Portobello Burgers

**Ingredients**
Coconut oil (1/2 tablespoon)
Oregano (1 teaspoon)
Portobello mushroom caps (2)
Garlic (1 clove)
Salt
Black pepper
Dijon mustard (1 tablespoon)
Cheddar cheese (1/4 cup)
Beef/bison (6 oz.)

**Directions**
1. Heat griddle and combine spices and oil in a bowl.
2. Remove gills from mushrooms and place into marinade until needed.
3. Add beef, cheese, salt, mustard and pepper in another bowl and mix to combine; form into a patty.
4. Place marinated caps onto grill and cook for 8 minutes until thoroughly heated. Place patty onto grill and cook on each side for 5 minutes.
5. Take 'buns' from grill and top with burger and any other toppings you choose.
6. Serve.

Servings: 1

**Nutrition Facts (per serving)**
Calories 735
Net Carbs 4g
Fats 48g
Protein 60g
Fiber 4g

# Chicken and Broccoli filled Zucchini

### Ingredients
Butter (2 tablespoons)
Broccoli (1 cup)
Sour cream (2 tablespoons)
Zucchini (10 oz.)-2
Cheddar cheese (3 oz., shredded)
Rotisserie chicken (6 oz., shredded)
Green onion (1 stalk)
Salt
Black pepper

### Directions
1. Set oven to 400 °F.
2. Slice zucchinis in half lengthwise and use spoons to remove cores. Melt butter and pour equally into each zucchini shell. Add black pepper and salt and bake for 20 minutes.
3. Chop broccoli and place into a bowl with sour cream and chicken. Fill zucchini boats with chicken mixture and top with cheese.
4. Bake for 15 minutes more or until golden.
5. Serve topped with green onion.

Servings: 2

### Nutrition Facts (per serving)
Calories 476.5
Net Carbs 5g
Fats 34g
Protein 30 g
Fiber 3g

# Super-Fast Egg Drop Soup

## Ingredients
Chicken broth (1 ½ cups)
Butter (1 tablespoon)
Chili garlic paste (1 teaspoon)
Chicken bouillon (1/2 cube)
Eggs (2)

## Directions
1. Add butter to pan, heat until it melts then add broth and bouillon
2. Bring to a boil and add chili paste, stir to combine and remove from flame.
3. Beat eggs in a bowl and add to broth, stir and put aside for a few minutes.
4. Serve.

Servings: 2

## Nutrition Facts (per serving)
Calories 279
Net Carbs 2.5g
Fats 23g
Protein 12g

# Salmon Salad in Avocado Cups

**Ingredients**

1 medium-sized salmon fillet
1 pc. Shallot, diced
¼ cup mayo
½ juice of lime
2 tsp. Fresh dill, chopped
1 tbsp. ghee
1 large avocado, sliced in half and pitted
salt and pepper to taste

**Directions**

1. Preheat oven at 400F
2. Place the salmon fillet on a baking sheet and drizzle it with ghee and juice of lime. Season with salt and pepper and place in the oven to cook for 20-25 minutes.
3. When done, allow the salmon to cook for a few minutes and shred using a fork.
4. Place the salmon in a bowl, add the diced shallot, and mix well.
5. Add the dill and mayo to the salmon mixture and combine well. Set aside.
6. Remove the insides of the avocado halves making sure that the skin is still intact to make cups.
7. Mash the avocado meat in a bowl and then add to the salmon mixture. Combine well.
8. Transfer the avocado and tuna salad back to the avocado cups and serve.

Servings: 2

**Nutrition Facts (per serving)**
Calories: 463
Net Carbs: 6.4g
Fat: 35g
Protein: 27g

170

# Cheesy Hotdog Pockets

**Ingredients**

2 pcs. beef hot dogs

2 thick sticks of quick-melt cheese (or mozzarella)

4 slices of bacon

1/8 tsp. garlic powder

1/8 tsp. onion powder

salt and pepper to taste

**Directions**

1. Preheat oven at 400F
2. Cut the hotdogs lengthwise to create slits.
3. Insert the cheese sticks in the hotdog and then wrap the bacon with to the beef hotdog. Secure the bacon using a toothpick.
4. Transfer the hotdogs on a baking sheet lined with foil and flavor with garlic and onion powder.
5. Place in the oven to cook for 40 minutes or until the hotdogs turns golden brown and the cheese is melted,
6. Serve with a veggie salad on the side.

**Nutrition Facts** (per serving)

Calories: 378

Net Carbs: 0.3 g

Fat: 35g

Protein: 17g

# Beef Shred Salad

**Ingredients**
2 cups beef, shredded
1 yellow pepper, sliced thin lengthwise
1 white onion, sliced lengthwise
6 pcs. butter lettuce
2 tsp. mayo
1/8 tsp. chili flakes

**Directions**
1. Place the butter lettuces on a serving plate. Spread mayo on the lettuce and top with the shredded beef.
2. Place pepper slices and onions on top and season with chili flakes.
3. Serve as it is or rolled.

**Nutrition Facts** (per serving)
Calories: 338
Net Carbs: 2.4
Fat: 25g
Protein: 24g

# Spicy Chicken Thighs

**Ingredients**

2 lb. chicken thighs
¼ cup ghee or olive oil
½ tsp. garlic powder
½ tsp. paprika
½ tsp. cumin, ground
¼ tsp. cayenne
¼ tsp. coriander, ground
1/8 tsp. cinnamon, ground
1/8 tsp. ginger powder
1 tsp. salt
1 tsp. yellow curry

**Directions**

1. Preheat oven at 425F.
2. In a small bowl mix all the spices to create a dry rub.
3. Pat dry the chicken using a kitchen paper towel and place on a baking sheet lined with greased parchment paper.
4. Generously brush the chicken with ghee or olive oil.
5. Rub the spices to the chicken thighs making sure that you cover every side.
6. Place the chicken in the oven to cook for 50 minutes.
7. Let it cool before serving.

**Nutrition Facts** (per serving)
Calories: 227
Net Carbs: .6g
Fat: 20g
Protein: 21g

# Spring Roll in a Bowl

**Ingredients**

500g pork mince
2 cups cabbage, shredded finely
2 cup grated carrot
2 cups grated baby marrows
1 cup mushrooms
4 tbsp. coconut Oil
1/2 cup soya sauce
1 cup chicken stock
2 tsp. vinegar
5 cloves garlic, minced
4 tsp. grated ginger
4 finely sliced spring onions
½ cup toasted sesame seeds
1 hard-boiled egg, chopped

**Directions**

1.  Heat the coconut oil and fry the garlic, spring onions, ginger.
2.  Add the pork mince and brown.
3.  Add the cabbage and carrot to the pot and toss to combine. Stir in the soy sauce.
4.  Cover and cook until the vegetables are soft, about 15 minutes.
5.  Dish up; add chopped hard-boiled egg over each of the bowls.
6.  Garnish with sesame seeds once you have dished up.

**Nutrition Facts** (per serving)
Calories: 80
Net Carbs: 5g
Fat: 5g
Protein: 3g

# Green Salad

**(This salad is the salad that is referred to across other meals)**

## Ingredients
1 cup green beans, steamed lightly
1 cup broccoli florets, steamed lightly
1 small tomato, finely sliced
1 cup lettuce
1 round feta
¼ cup toasted sunflower seeds, roasted
1 hard-boiled egg, chopped

For dressing:
1 tbsp. olive oil
Salt and pepper to taste
juice from ½ lemon

## Directions
1. Place all the vegetables in a salad bowl.
2. Crumble the feta and sprinkle it along with the roasted pumpkin seeds and egg on top of the salad.
3. In a small bowl, pour the olive oil, add lemon juice, then add salt and pepper, and whisk together. Drizzle this dressing on top of the salad.
4. Toss gently before serving.

## Nutrition Facts (per serving)
Calories: 45
Net Carbs: 3g
Fat: 3g
Protein: 1g

# Greek Salad

**Ingredients**
50g Grilled Chicken Breast
2 cups lettuce
10 Olives
½ Round Feta
5 Cherry Tomatoes
¼ Cucumber
1Tblsp Olive Oil
1tsp. Lemon juice

**Directions**
1.  Place all ingredients into a bowl, mix and enjoy!

# Bacon, Lettuce, Tomato Salad

**Ingredients**

1 cup of lettuce
1 spring onion
1 tomato
¼ cup toasted pumpkin seeds
grated boiled egg
sliced avocado
4 rashes of crispy bacon (crumbled)

For dressing:
1 Tbsp. apple cider vinegar
1 tsp. lemon juice
½ a finely crushed clove of garlic
1 Tbsp. Olive oil and some finely crushed fresh ginger (optional)

**Directions**

1. In a large bowl combine salad ingredients
2. This can all be done at home and taken to work.

For dressing:

1. In a separate container mix dressing ingredients
2. Allow the dressing to sit for a few hours.

Pour the dressing over the salad when you are ready to eat.

# Broccoli Salad

### Ingredients
1 cup broccoli
2 medium celery stalks
1/2 cup mushroom pieces (fried)
1/4 cup Cherry tomatoes
1Tblsp olive oil
2 cups Lettuce
1Tblsp Balsamic Vinegar
125ml pumpkin seeds roasted dry in a pan.

### Directions
1. Place all ingredients into a bowl, mix and enjoy!

# Tuna/Smoked Salmon Salad

### Ingredients
1 Tin Tuna in Water/100g Smoked Salmon
1 Hard Boiled Egg
½ Avo
1 Cup Green Beans (Steamed)
5 Cherry Tomatoes
1 Tbsp. Red Onion
½ Cup Celery

### Directions
1. Place all ingredients into a bowl, mix and enjoy!

## Avo & Tuna Lettuce Wraps

In a medium bowl, combine all ingredients for tuna salad. Mix with a fork. Refrigerate. To assemble, spoon tuna mixture into lettuce leaves. Top with avocado and tomato.

# Warm Chicken Salad

### Ingredients
1. Roast 2 medium chicken thighs in the oven the night before and remove meat from bones (eat skin whilst warm).
2. Reheat Chicken the following day and add to salad

# Hearty Salad

### Ingredients
1 Hard Boiled Egg grated
2 slices of country ham, finely sliced
30g cheddar cheese
1 tomato finely diced
2Tblsp Mayo
1 cup finely sliced crispy lettuce
2 spring onions finely chopped
½ green pepper finely chopped

### Directions
1. Combine all the ingredients and then add the mayo and mix.

# Crunchy Chicken Waldorf Salad

### Ingredients
150ml full cream plain yogurt
1Tblsp Mayonnaise
2 teaspoons lemon juice
1/4 teaspoon salt
50g chopped cooked chicken breast
½ medium green apple, finely diced
1 cup finely sliced celery
1/2 cup chopped walnuts, toasted.

### Directions
1. Whisk mayonnaise, yogurt, lemon juice and salt in a large bowl.
2. Add chicken, apple, celery and 1/4 cup walnuts.
3. Stir to coat well. Serve topped with the remaining 1/4 cup walnuts.

# Spinach Cheese & Bacon Log

**Ingredients**

Cheddar cheese (2 ½ cups, shredded)

Chipotle seasoning (2 tablespoons)

Bacon (30 slices)

Mrs. Dash seasoning (2 teaspoons)

Spinach (5 cups)

**Directions**
1. Set oven to 375 F.
2. Place bacon in a weaving pattern on a baking sheet lined with foil and season with spices.
3. Top bacon with cheese leaving a 1 inch space all around the edge. Add spinach and push it down and roll the bacon together into a log.
4. Sprinkle with salt and place into oven for 60 minutes.
5. Cool for 15 minutes and slice.
6. Serve.

Servings: 5

**Nutrition Facts (per serving)**

Calories 432

Net Carbs 3g

Fats 38.2g

Protein 32.8 g

Fiber 3g

# Beef Sausage, Bacon & Broccoli Casserole

**Ingredients**
500 g beef sausage
1/2 head of broccoli
8 slices of bacon
Cream (1/2 cups)
Dijon mustard (1 tablespoon)
100 g grated cheddar cheese

**Directions**
1. Preheat oven to 350F
2. Slice the sausage and place in a small baking dish.
3. Slice the bacon and add to the sausage.
4. Break the broccoli into florets and arrange between the meat.
5. Mix the cream and mustard in a bowl and pour it all over the casserole, then top with the cheese.
6. Bake in the oven for 35 minutes.

**Nutrition Facts (per serving)**
Calories: 300
Net Carbs: 3g
Fat: 25g
Protein: 20g

# Zucchini Stuffed with Chicken & Broccoli

**Ingredients**
Butter (2 tablespoons)
Broccoli (1 cup)
Sour cream (2 tablespoons)
Zucchini (10 oz.)-2
Cheddar cheese (3 oz., shredded)
Rotisserie chicken (6 oz., shredded)
Green onion (1 stalk)
Salt
Black pepper

**Directions**
1. Set oven to 400°F.
2. Slice zucchinis in half lengthwise and use spoons to remove cores. Melt butter and pour equally into each zucchini shell. Add black pepper and salt and bake for 20 minutes.
3. Chop broccoli and place into a bowl with sour cream and chicken. Fill zucchini boats with chicken mixture and top with cheese.
4. Bake for 15 minutes more or until golden.
5. Serve topped with green onion.

Servings: 2

**Nutrition Facts (per serving)**
Calories 476.5
Net Carbs 5g
Fats 34g
Protein 30 g
Fiber 3g

# Beef Pumpkin Chili

**Ingredients**

2 lbs. ground beef
1 can (15 oz.) pumpkin puree
1 Tbsp. pumpkin pie spice
3 cups 100% tomato juice
3 tomatoes, diced
1 red bell pepper
1 yellow onion
2 tsp. cumin
1 Tbsp. chili powder
2 tsp. cayenne pepper
ghee or coconut oil

**Directions**

1. In a large frying pan greased with ghee or coconut oil, brown the meat over medium heat.
2. Chop the onion and pepper and add into the pot with the meat. Cook 3-5 minutes or until the onions become translucent.
3. Add in the rest of the ingredients and let simmer on LOW for 30 minutes.
4. Season chili with salt and pepper to taste and cook for another 30 minutes.
5. Serve hot.

Servings: 8

Cooking Time: 1 hour and 20 minutes

**Nutrition Facts (per serving)**

Calories 354, 83
Fat 25,24g
Fiber 2,14g
Sugar 5,5g
Protein 21,87g

# Dinner Recipes

# Beef Cabbage Parsley Soup

**Ingredients**

1 lb. beef shank
1/2 head cabbage, chopped
6 tsp. fresh parsley (chopped)
2 zucchini, cubed
1 tomato, quartered
1 onion, chopped
4 cloves garlic, minced
1 Tbsp. salt
1/4 tsp. ground cumin
2 Tbsp. fresh lime juice

**Directions**

1. In a large pot over low heat combine the beef, tomato, zucchini, onion, cabbage, garlic, 5 teaspoons parsley, salt and cumin.
2. Add water to cover and stir well. Cover lid and cook for 2 hours.
3. Remove lid, stir, and simmer for another 1 hour with lid off.
4. Just before eating, squeeze in fresh lime juice to taste and sprinkle with remaining parsley.
5. Serve hot.

Servings: 8

**Cooking Times**
Total Time: 2 hours and 5 minutes

**Nutrition Facts (per serving)**
Calories 129
Fat 2,35g
Carbs 13,28g
Fiber 2,08g
Protein 14,11g

# Boneless Lamb Stew

### Ingredients
2 lbs. boneless lamb meat, cubed
1 cup red onion, chopped
2 whole celery stalks, diced
4 cloves garlic, minced
1 cup tomato juice
2 Tbsp. extra virgin coconut oil
1 cup lime juice (freshly squeezed)
1 bay leaf
1 tsp. ground cinnamon
1 tsp. ground nutmeg
Fresh parsley, chopped for topping
Sea salt and freshly ground black pepper, to taste

### Directions
1. Put the lamb in a glass bowl and season with the salt, pepper, cinnamon, and nutmeg. Place in refrigerator for up to 24 hours.
2. In a large casserole, heat the coconut oil over medium heat. Add pieces of lamb and brown on all sides.
3. Once browned, add the onion, garlic and celery. Cook for about five minutes, stirring often, until vegetables start to soften.
4. Add the tomato juice, lime juice and bay leaf; stir till mixture begins to boil.
5. Reduce the heat to low and cook for about 2 hours.
6. Serve hot with fresh chopped parsley.

Servings: 6

Cooking Times
Total Time: 2 hours and 10 minutes

### Nutrition Facts (per serving)
Calories 250
Fat 11,82g
Carbs 6,86g
Fiber 1,67g
Protein 21,68g

186

# Baked Cheesy Meatballs

**Ingredients**
1 lb. ground beef (lean)
2 white onion
1 cup grated Cheddar cheese
4 oz. Gruyere cheese
1 egg
1.5 tsp. nutmeg
1.5 tsp. allspice
sea salt and freshly black pepper to taste
butter for greasing

**Directions**
1. Preheat oven to 350F.
2. In a greased frying pan, sauté onions until translucent. Remove from heat, and let cool.
3. In a food processor mince the Gruyere cheese. Set aside.
4. In a mixing bowl, whisk egg with grated Cheddar cheese. Add the spices, salt, and pepper and mix.
5. Add in onions and Gruyere cheese. Mix well until smooth.
6. Add the beef and mix until all ingredients are combined well.
7. Divide meat mixture and roll each piece into a ball.
8. Place the meatballs on a cookie sheet, and bake in preheated oven about 20 minutes. Serve hot.

Servings: 6

**Cooking Times**
Total Time: 35 minutes

**Nutrition Facts (per serving)**
Calories 385
Fat 29,05g
Carbs 4,79g
Fiber 0,91g
Protein 25,25g

# Chicken & Endive Casserole

**Ingredients**

1 endive head, cut into wide strips

1 1/2 lbs. skinless boneless chicken thighs

1 Tbsp. dried oregano

2 cups chopped onions

4 celery stalks, chopped

4 garlic cloves, chopped

1 cup diced tomatoes in juice

2 Tbsp. olive oil

8 cups water

**Directions**

1. In a large saucepan heat oil over medium-high heat.
2. Sprinkle the chicken with salt, pepper, and oregano. Add chicken in a saucepan. Mix in onions, celery and garlic. Sauté until vegetables begin to soften, about 4-5minutes.
3. Stir in tomatoes. Add broth; bring to boil. Reduce heat to medium; simmer until vegetables and chicken are tender, about 15 minutes.
4. Add endive hearts; simmer until wilted, about 3 minutes. Season with salt and pepper.
5. Ladle into bowls and serve hot.

Servings: 6

**Cooking Times**

Total Time: 40 minutes

**Nutrition Facts (per serving)**

Calories 144,

Fat 7,21g

Carbs 9,94g

Fiber 2,05g

Protein 9,89g

# Creamy Smoked Turkey Salad with Almonds

**Ingredients**

Salad ingredients:
2 cups diced, cooked smoked turkey breast
1/4 cup sliced almonds
1/2 cup diced celery
1/4 cup sliced green onions
1/4 cup shredded cabbage

Dressing ingredients:
4 oz. mayonnaise
2 oz. sour cream
2 drops sweet liquid Splenda
1 tsp. curry powder
Salt and pepper to taste

**Directions**
1.  In a bowl, combine sour cream and mayonnaise and whisk until smooth. Add the spices and continue to whisk until smooth.
2.  In a big bowl, combine all salad ingredients and the dressing and toss well. Serve and enjoy!

**Note:** *You can make the dressing a day ahead of time, and store in the fridge to let the flavors meld.*

Servings: 4

Cooking Times
Total Time: 10 minutes

**Nutrition Facts (per serving)**
Calories 235
Fat 17,65g
Carbs 10,99g
Fiber 1,65g
Protein 9,84g

# Herb Baked Salmon Fillets

### Ingredients
2 lbs. salmon fillets
1/2 cup chopped fresh mushrooms
1/2 cup chopped green onions
4 oz. butter
4 Tbsp. coconut oil
1/2 cup tamari soy sauce
1 tsp. minced garlic
1/4 tsp. thyme
1/2 tsp. rosemary
1/4 tsp. tarragon
1/2 tsp. ground ginger
1/2 tsp. basil
1 tsp. oregano leaves

### Directions
1. Preheat oven to 350 degrees F. Line a large baking pan with foil.
2. Cut salmon filet in pieces. Put the salmon into the Ziploc bag with the tamari sauce, sesame oil and spices sauce mixture. Refrigerate the salmon and marinade it for 4 hours.
3. Put the salmon in a baking pan and bake fillets for 10-15 minutes.
4. Melt the butter. Add the chopped fresh mushrooms and green onion to it, and mix. Remove the salmon from the oven, and pour the butter mixture over the salmon fillets, making sure each fillet gets covered. Bake for about 10 minutes more. Serve immediately.

Servings: 6
### Cooking Times
Inactive Time: 4 hours
Total Time: 35 minutes

### Nutrition Facts (per serving)
Calories 449
Fat 34,11g
Carbs 2,77g
Fiber 0,72g
Protein 33,19g

# Butternut Squash Soup

**Ingredients**

3 lbs. butternut squash
4 cloves garlic, minced
1 cup yellow onion, sliced
1 cup coconut milk
2 tsp. olive oil
1 bay leaf
2 cup water
1/2 tsp. salt and pepper (per taste)
coconut oil or olive oil for greasing

**Directions**

1. Preheat oven to 450° F.
2. On a greased baking sheet, place the squash and onion with half oil and salt. Roast in a single layer about 25-30 minutes.
3. Transfer the vegetables to a large saucepan with olive oil and cook over HIGH heat for 3-5 minutes. Stir often.
4. Add garlic and cook for another 30 seconds. Add the water, bay leaf and coconut milk; bring to a boil.
5. Reduce heat to MEDIUM-LOW, cover and simmer for 10 minutes more.
6. At the end, remove bay leaf and transfer squash mixture to a blender. Puree until smooth. Add salt and pepper to taste.
7. Ladle to bowls and serve hot.

Servings: 10

**Cooking Times**
Total Time: 55 minutes

**Nutrition Facts (per serving)**
Calories 120
Fat 7,12g
Carbs 12,74g
Fiber 2,3g
Protein 3,48g

# Creamy Chicken Salad

**Ingredients**
Salad ingredients
2 cups diced, cooked chicken
1/2 cup sliced green onion
1/4 cup parsley, chopped
1/2 cup diced celery
Dressing ingredients
4 oz. mayonnaise
2 oz. blue cream cheese, softened
1 tsp. dried tarragon
1/2 tsp. dried thyme
salt and pepper to taste

**Directions**
1. In a bowl, whisk cream cheese and mayonnaise until smooth.
2. Add the spices and continue to whisk.
3. Combine the salad ingredients and add dressing to taste, mixing to coat all the ingredients.
4. Serve immediately.

Servings: 4

**Cooking Times**
Total Time: 10 minutes

**Nutrition Facts (per serving)**
Calories 250
Fat 12,23g
Carbs 9,77g
Fiber 0,78g
Protein 24,74g

# Duck Breast with Balsamic Vinegar

**Ingredients**

1 lb. duck breasts

4 Tbsp. duck fat (or lark)

4 green onions (chopped)

1 tsp. fresh ginger grated

1/2 Tbsp. lime juice

Marjoram to taste

2 Tbsp. coconut oil

2 Tbsp. apple cider vinegar

salt and freshly ground pepper to taste

**Directions**

1. In a frying pan add 1 tablespoon coconut oil and add the duck breast. Sauté it at high heat about 3-4 minutes.
2. In a deep saucepan add the duck fat, and add the duck meat. Cook for 3 hours about. Add the chopped green onions in the last 30 minutes of the cooking process.
3. Remove green onion and duck breast from the heat, and place them in a separate dish to cool down. Sprinkle the marjoram, balsamic vinegar and the lime juice. Serve hot.

Servings: 4

**Nutrition Facts (per serving)**

Calories 471,

Fat 46,68g

Carbs 2,76g

Fiber 0,42g

Protein 10,11g

# Hot Mexican Meatballs

### Ingredients
1 lb. ground beef (92% lean)
4 oz. white onion, minced
4 oz. Monterey Jack cheese with spicy peppers
1 Tbsp. butter
3 cloves garlic
1 1 tsp. chili powder
1 1 tsp. ground cumin
1 tsp. ground coriander
1 egg
sea salt and freshly ground pepper to taste

### Directions
1. Preheat oven to 350 degrees.
2. In a frying pan, sauté onions in butter until translucent. Set aside
3. Shred and mince the Monterey Jack cheese with spicy peppers. Set aside.
4. In a mixing bowl, whisk egg with ricotta cheese. Add the spices, salt, and pepper and mix.
5. Add onions and minced Monterey Jack cheese with spicy peppers. Mix well.
6. Add beef and mix until all ingredients are combined.
7. Roll the meat mix into a ball.
8. Place the meatballs on a cookie sheet, and bake about 20 minutes.
9. Serve hot.

Servings: 6

Cooking Times
Total Time: 35 minutes

### Nutrition Facts (per serving)
Calories 321
Fat 25,25g
Carbs 2,94g
Fiber 0,9g
Protein 19,54g

194

# Lamb Cutlets with Garlic Sauce

**Ingredients**
4 lbs. lamb cutlets
1 small head of garlic, cloves peeled
2 Tbsp. apple cider vinegar
1/2 cup water
1/4 cup extra virgin olive oil
pinch salt and black ground pepper to taste

**Directions**
1. Crush the garlic cloves thoroughly in a mortar. In a bowl, add the vinegar and water and mix it well with the crushed garlic. Set aside.
2. In a large frying pan, pour the olive oil and fry the lamb cutlets until nicely brown.
3. Add the garlic mixture and let it cook gently for about 10 minutes.
4. Shake the frying pan to spread the garlic mixture evenly over the lamb.
5. Season with salt and black pepper to taste. Serve.

Servings: 10

**Cooking Times**
Total Time: 40 minutes

**Nutrition Facts (per serving)**
Calories 416
Fat 28,76g
Carbs 0,16g
Fiber 0,01g
Protein 36,68g

# Almond Bread

**Ingredients**

2 eggs
1 cup almond butter, unsalted
3/4 cup almond flour
1 Tbsp. cinnamon
1 tsp. pure vanilla extract
1/4 tsp. baking soda
2 Tbsp. liquid Stevia
1/2 tsp. sea salt

**Directions**

1. Preheat oven to 340F degrees.
2. In a deep bowl whisk eggs, almond butter, honey, Stevia and vanilla. Add in salt, cinnamon and baking soda. Stir until all ingredients are well combined.
3. Pour dough in a greased baking pan. Bake for 12-15 minutes.
4. Once ready, let cool on a wire rack. Slice and serve.

Servings: 8

**Cooking Times**
Total Time: 25 minutes

**Nutrition Facts (per serving)**
Calories 208
Fat 16,7g
Carbs 7,64g
Fiber 3,63g
Protein 7,7g

# Slow Cooker Buffalo Chicken

## Ingredients

3 Tbsp. butter

6 frozen chicken breasts

1 bottle of your favorite cayenne peppers sauce

1 cup of your favorite garlic sauce

## Directions

1. Put the chicken in the bottom of your Slow Cooker. Pour the hot sauce over chicken and sprinkle ranch over top
2. Cover the lid and cook on LOW for 6 hours.
3. Once ready, add butter, and cook on LOW uncovered for one hour more. Serve hot.

Servings: 4

Cooking Time: 6 hours and 5 minutes

## Nutrition Facts (per serving)

Calories 517

Fat 18,41g

Carbs 2,26g

Fiber 0,37g

Protein 80,37g

# Spiced Kale "Meatballs"

**Ingredients**
4 Tbsp. olive oil
1 cup almond flour
1 bunch of kale leaves
1 green chili, chopped
1/4 tsp. red chili powder
1/4 tsp. turmeric powder
1 tsp. cumin seed powder
1/4 tsp. ginger, minced
black salt or salt as per taste
1 tsp. cooking soda or baking soda (optional)
water for batter

**Directions**
1. In a bowl, mix all the ingredients together.
2. Combine and knead the batter with your finger. The consistency should be nor too thick nor too thin. Make a kale "meatballs".
3. Heat oil in a frying pan. Place a kale "meatballs" in the hot oil one by one.
4. Fry few at a time don't cluster with too many. When they get golden color from one side, turn and cook from another side.
5. Remove the fries with slotted spoon and place over absorbent napkins.
6. Serve hot.

Servings: 8

**Cooking Times**
Total Time: 25 minutes

**Nutrition Facts (per serving)**
Calories 125
Fat 6,24g
Carbs 13,01g
Fiber 4,85g
Protein 6,04g

# Spinach Soup with Almonds and Parmesan

**Ingredients**
1 lb. baby spinach leaves
1 leek
1 zucchini (medium)
1/4 cup parmesan cheese (grated)
4 Tbsp. olive oil
4 cups water
15 almond shivers
salt and black ground pepper to taste

**Directions**
1. Wash the leek and cut it into thick slices.
2. Heat the olive oil in a saucepan and cook the zucchini and leek for about 2-3 minutes.
3. Add the cleaned spinach leaves, water and a pinch of salt. Bring to the boil and let it simmer for 15 minutes.
4. Remove from the heat and place the vegetables in a food processor. Blend into a very smooth soup.
5. In a frying pan, toast the almonds. Pour the soup into bowls, sprinkle with some Parmesan cheese on top and toasted almonds.
6. Serve.

Servings: 6

**Cooking Times**
Total Time: 45 minutes

**Nutrition Facts (per serving)**
Calories 63
Fat 3,04g
Carbs 5,94g
Fiber 2,47g
Protein 4,84g

# Stuffed Avocado with Tuna

## Ingredients

2 ripe avocados, halved and pitted
1 can (15 oz.) solid white tuna packed in water, drained
2 Tbsp. mayonnaise
3 green onions, thinly sliced
1 Tbsp. cayenne paprika
1 red bell pepper, chopped
1 Tbsp. balsamic vinegar
1 pinch garlic salt and black pepper to taste

## Directions

1. In a bowl, toss together tuna, mayonnaise, cayenne pepper, green onions, red pepper, and balsamic vinegar.
2. Season with pepper and salt, and then pack the avocado halves with the tuna mixture.
3. Ready! Serve and enjoy!

Servings: 4

## Cooking Times

Total Time: 20 minutes

## Nutrition Facts (per serving)

Calories 233
Fat 17,77g
Carbs 13,87g
Fiber 6,98g
Protein 7,41g

# Light Cabbage Soup

**Ingredients**
2 1/2 cups chopped cabbage
4 garlic cloves, minced
1 Tbsp. tomato paste
1 onion, chopped
1/2 cup parsnip, chopped
1/2 cup cauliflower florets
1/2 cup chopped zucchini
1/2 tsp. basil
1/2 tsp. oregano
Salt and black pepper, to taste
4 cups water
olive oil for sautéing

**Directions**
1. In a frying pan, sauté onions, parsnip and garlic for 5 minutes.
2. Add in water, tomato paste, cabbage, cauliflower, basil, oregano and salt and pepper to taste.
3. Simmer for about 5-10 minutes until all vegetables are tender. Add the zucchini and simmer for another 5 minutes.
4. Serve hot.

Servings: 4

**Cooking Times**
Total Time: 35 minutes

**Nutrition Facts (per serving)**
Calories 80
Fat 3,08g
Carbs 9,69g
Fiber 3,04g
Protein 4,62g

# Oriental Shrimp Soup

## Ingredients

12 oz. fresh shrimp, peeled and deveined
1 cup zucchini (medium, sliced)
1 onion, chopped
2 cloves garlic, minced
1 Tbsp. ginger, minced
1 pinch crushed red pepper
2 quarts water
1 cup celery (chopped)
2 cups cauliflower florets
2 Tbsp. soy sauce
1/4 tsp. ground black pepper
2 tsp. olive oil

## Directions

1. In a large saucepan with over medium heat cook onion, garlic, ginger and crushed red pepper for 2 minutes.
2. Pour in water, cauliflower florets and celery and bring to a boil. Reduce heat, cover and simmer 5 minutes.
3. Stir in zucchini and shrimp, season with salt and pepper to taste; cover and cook 5 - 7 minutes.
4. Stir in soy sauce and pepper and serve.

Servings: 8

## Cooking Times

Total Time: 25 minutes

## Nutrition Facts (per serving)

Calories 107
Fat 3,08g
Carbs 7,12g
Fiber 1,6g
Protein 12,08g

# Slow Cooker Beef with Dried Herbs

**Ingredients**
1 1/2 lbs. lean beef
2 celery ribs
1 cup beef broth
2 Tbsp. amaranth flour
2 Tbsp. almond butter
2 Tbsp. olive oil
1 tsp. mustard
2 Tbsp. fresh lemon juice
4 Tbsp. chopped parsley
salt, pepper, dried thyme, dried marjoram

**Directions**
1. In a bowl, toss the beef with the amaranth flour. Heat the butter and oil in a skillet; add the beef and cook, stirring, until browned.
2. In a slow cooker combine the browned beef with remaining ingredients, except lemon juice and parsley.
3. Cover and cook on LOW for 6 to 8 hours.
4. Once ready, stir in lemon juice and parsley and serve hot.

Servings: 6

**Cooking Times**
Total Time: 8 hours

**Nutrition Facts (per serving)**
Calories 387
Fat 31,96g
Carbs 2,56g
Fiber 0,2g
Protein 20,96g

# Zucchini Soup with Crunchy Cured Ham

**Ingredients**
2 leeks (white part only)
12 ounces zucchinis
10 ounces summer squash
3 Tbsp. virgin olive oil
5 cups water
salt
2 slices cured ham
black pepper

**Directions**
1. Cut the leeks into thin slices and chop the zucchinis and summer squash into cubes.
2. In a large saucepan, heat the olive oil and add the leeks. Cook the leeks until they are soft, stirring gently.
3. Add in the chopped zucchinis and summer squash and cook them for about 5 minutes.
4. Add in water and bring to the boil for about 15 minutes.
5. Blend or process the soup in batches until smooth.
6. Season the soup to taste.
7. In a frying pan cook striped ham until crispy.
8. Divide the soup amongst the serving bowls and sprinkle with the crunchy ham strips and some black pepper.
9. Serve hot.

Servings: 4

**Cooking Times**
Total Time: 45 minutes

**Nutrition Facts (per serving)**
Calories 84
Fat 1,89g
Carbs 8,75g
Fiber 1,52g
Protein 8,54g

# Salmon with a Walnut Crust

**Ingredients**
Walnuts (1/2 cup)
Dijon mustard (1/2 tablespoon)
Salmon filets (6 oz.)-2
Salt
Maple syrup (2 tablespoons, sugar free)
Dill (1/4 teaspoon)
Olive oil (1 tablespoon)

**Directions**
1. Set oven to 350˚F.
2. Put mustard, syrup and walnuts into a processor and pulse until mixture is pasty.
3. Heat oil in a pot and place the skin side down in the pan and sear for 3 minutes.
4. Top it with walnut blend and place into a lined baking dish.
5. Bake for 8 minutes.
6. Serve.

Servings: 2

**Nutrition Facts (per serving)**
Calories 373
Fats 43g
Protein 20 g
Fiber 1g

# Cheeseburger Casserole

**Ingredients**

Bacon (3 slices)
Cauliflower (1 ¼ cups)
Garlic powder (1/2 teaspoon)
Ketchup (2 tablespoons, no sugar)
Mayonnaise (2 tablespoons)
Cheddar cheese (4 oz.)
Ground beef (1 lb.)
Almond flour (1/2 cup)
Psyllium Husk Powder (1 tablespoon)
Onion powder (1/2 teaspoon)
Dijon mustard (1 tablespoon)
Eggs (3)
Salt
Black pepper

**Directions**

1. Set oven to 350 °F.
2. Place cauliflower into a processor and pulse until fine like rice. Add remaining dry ingredients except cheese.
3. Add beef and bacon in processor until combined and pasty.
4. Heat skillet and cook meat for 8 minutes then add to dry ingredients in bowl along with half of cheese. Stir to combine and line a baking dish with parchment paper.
5. Press mixture into dish and top with leftover cheese. Bake for 30 minutes on top rack.
6. Take from heat, cool and slice.
7. Serve.

Servings: 6

**Nutrition Facts (per serving)**

Calories 478
Net Carbs 3.6g
Fats 35.5g
Protein 32.2 g
Fiber 3.3g

# Curried Coconut Chicken Fingers

**Ingredients**
Chicken thighs (24 oz., boneless with skin)
Pork rinds (1/2 cup, crushed)
Curry powder (2 teaspoons)
Garlic powder (1/4 teaspoon)
Salt & Black pepper
Egg (1)
Coconut (1/2 cup, shredded, unsweetened)
Coriander (1/2 teaspoon)
Onion powder (1/4 teaspoon)

For Dipping Sauce:
Sour cream (1/4 cup)
Mango extract (1 ½ teaspoons)
Garlic powder (1/2 teaspoon)
Cayenne powder (1/4 teaspoon)
Mayonnaise (1/4 cup)
Ketchup (2 tablespoons, sugar free)
Red pepper flakes (1 ½ teaspoons)
Ground ginger (1/2 teaspoon)
Liquid Stevia (7 drops)

**Directions**
1. Set oven to 400°F.
2. Beat egg in a bowl and slice chicken into strips.
3. Combine spices, pork rind and coconut in another bowl. Coat with egg and then in dry mix.
4. Place onto a lined baking sheet and bake for 15 minutes and turn over; bake for an additional 20 minutes. Combine all ingredients for dipping sauce in a bowl and serve with chicken.

Servings: 6

**Nutrition Facts (per serving)**
Calories 494
Net Carbs 2.1g
Fats 39.4g
Protein 29.4 g
Fiber 1.2g

# Slow Cooker Lamb Curry & Spinach

**Ingredients**
Coconut or olive oil (1/3 cup)
3 copped yellow onions
4 cloves garlic, peeled and minced
2cm piece of ginger, peeled and grated
Ground cumin (2 teaspoons)
Cayenne pepper (1 1/2 teaspoons).
Ground turmeric (1 1/2 teaspoons).
Beef stock, high quality (2 cups)
Leg of lamb, cut into 2cm cubes (53 oz.)
Salt
Baby spinach (6 cups)
Plain full-fat yogurt (2 cups)

**Directions**
1.  In a large frying pan over medium-high heat, warm oil. Add onions and garlic, and sauté until golden, about 5 minutes. Stir in ginger, cumin, cayenne, and turmeric and sauté until fragrant, or for about 30 seconds.
2.  Pour in broth scraping up the browned bits on the bottom. When broth comes to a boil, remove pan from heat.
3.  Put lamb in a slow cooker, and sprinkle with 1 tbsp. salt. Add contents of frying pan. Cover and cook on high-heat setting for 4 hours or low-heat setting for 8 hours.
4.  Add baby spinach to pot and cook, stirring occasionally, until spinach is wilted, about 5 minutes. Just before serving, stir in 1 1/3 cups yogurt. Season to taste with salt.

Servings: 5

**Nutrition Facts (per serving)**
Calories- 304
Carbs- 5.5g
Protein- 32.85g
Fats- 16.32g

# Curried Madras Lamb

**Ingredients**
8 Fatty lamb chops
Coconut Milk (6 tablespoons)
2 cups water
Red Curry Paste (3 tablespoons)
Thai fish sauce (2 tablespoons)
Dried onion flakes (1 tablespoon)
Dried Thai or fresh red chilies (2 tablespoons)
Xylitol (1 tablespoon)
Ground cumin (1 tablespoon)
Ground coriander (1 tablespoon)
Ground cloves (1/8 teaspoon)
Ground nutmeg (1/8 teaspoon)
Ground ginger (1 tablespoon)

To Serve:
Coconut milk powder (2 tablespoons)
Red curry paste (1 tablespoons)
Xylitol (2 tablespoons)
1/4 cup cashews, roughly chopped
1/4 cup fresh cilantro, chopped

**Directions**
1.  Place the raw lamb chops in a large slow cooker.
2.  Add the 6 tbsp. coconut milk, water, 3 tbsp. red curry paste, fish sauce, onion flakes, chilies, 1 tbsp. Xylitol, cumin, coriander, cloves, nutmeg, and ginger. Cover and cook on high for about 5 hours (or low for 8).
3.  Just before serving, scoop out the meat to another dish. Then whisk into the sauce the 2 tbsp. coconut milk powder, 1 tbsp. curry paste, 2 tbsp. sweetener, and 1/4 tsp. xanthan gum (if using).
4.  Break the meat into pieces and stir into the sauce, along with the chopped cashews. Garnish with chopped coriander before serving

Servings: 5
**Nutrition Facts (per serving)**
Calories- 190
Carbs- 4g
Protein- 18g
Fats- 11g

# Seafood Stew

**Ingredients**
Olive oil (1 tablespoon)
2 onions, diced
4 stalks celery, chopped
4 garlic cloves, minced
Dried oregano (1 teaspoon)
Ground black pepper (1/2 teaspoon)
Tomato paste (1 tablespoon)
Flour (1 tablespoon)
3 cups chicken stock
1 can tomato, onion and chili mix
1 -2 cup tomato cocktail juice
4 chicken breasts cut into bite size pieces
2 packets mixed frozen seafood, you can add extra
mussels in at the end
2 peppers (red and green)
1 jalapeno pepper, chopped
1/4cup parsley, chopped
Chili powder (1 teaspoon)
1 pinch cayenne pepper
Butter (1 tablespoon)

**Directions**
1. In a large pan heat the olive oil and fry onions and celery
2. Add garlic, oregano, peppercorns.
3. Stir in tomato paste and almond flour and cook another minute.
4. Add chicken stock, tomatoes and tomato juice and bring to a boil. Continue to cook for about 3-5 more minutes. Remove from heat and transfer mixture to slow cooker.
5. Add chicken and stir to combine. Cover and cook on high for 3 hours or low for 6 hours. Stir in mixed bags of frozen and parsley. Cover and cook on high for 30 minutes

Servings: 5
**Nutrition Facts (per serving)**
Calories- 177
Carbs- 15g
Protein- 21g
Fats- 4g

# Slow Cooker Thai Fish Curry

**Ingredients**
Coconut oil (1 tablespoon)
Green Thai curry paste (1/2 tablespoons)
8-10 spring onions
2 garlic cloves, crushed
1 Thai red chili, deseeded if you like, and thinly sliced
Turmeric (1 teaspoon)
Chicken stock (160ml)
1½ cups coconut milk
2.5cm piece of fresh ginger, peeled and sliced
Xylitol (2 teaspoons)
Juice of 1 lime, plus extra to taste
Fish sauce (1 teaspoon)
700g boneless, skinless white fish, such as cod, hake or halibut cut into large chunks
freshly ground black pepper
chopped coriander leaves, to serve

**Directions**
1. Fry Spring onions, garlic and chilies then stir in green Thai Curry Paste and then sprinkle over the turmeric.
2. Add the stock, coconut milk, ginger, Xylitol and juice from a fresh lime and season with pepper. Bring to the boil, stirring to dissolve the paste and xylitol, and then pour the mixture into the slow cooker.
3. Cover the cooker with the lid and cook on HIGH for 1 hour until the flavors are well blended. Add the fish sauce, if using, and add a little more xylitol and fresh lime juice, if you like.
4. Switch the cooker to LOW. Add the fish, re-cover and cook until the fish is cooked through and flakes easily.
5. Sprinkle with coriander and lime zest and sliced red chilies.

Servings: 5

**Nutrition Facts (per serving)**
Calories 312
Carbs 20g
Protein 24g
Fats 15g

# Smoky Pork Cassoulet

### Ingredients
1 pack bacon, fried and then crumbled
Chopped onion (2 cups)
Dried thyme (1 teaspoon)
Dried rosemary (1/2 teaspoon)
3 garlic cloves, crushed
Salt (1/2 teaspoon)
Freshly ground black pepper (1/2 teaspoon)
2 cans diced tomatoes, drained
500g boneless pork loin roast, trimmed and cut into 2cm cubes
250g smoked sausage, cut into 1cm cubes
Finely shredded fresh Parmesan cheese (8 teaspoons)
Chopped fresh flat-leaf parsley (8 teaspoons)

### Directions
1. Fry bacon onion, thyme, rosemary, and garlic, then add salt, pepper, and tomatoes; bring to a boil.
2. Remove from heat.
3. Place all ingredients in the slow cooker, alternating the meat with the tomato sauce until finished. Cover and cook on low for 5 hours. Sprinkle with Parmesan cheese and parsley when cooked

Servings: 4

### Nutrition Facts (per serving)
Calories- 258
Carbs- 10.8g
Protein- 27g
Fats- 12.6g

# Sage and Orange Glazed Duck

**Ingredients**
Butter (2 tablespoons)
Swerve (1 tablespoon)
Sage (1/4 teaspoon)
Duck breast (6 oz.)
Heavy cream (1 tablespoon)
Orange extract (1/2 teaspoon)
Spinach (1 cup)

**Directions**
1. Use knife to score the skin of the duck and season with black pepper and salt.
2. Add Swerve and butter to a pot and cook until slightly golden then add extract and sage. Cook until butter has darkened.
3. In another pot, place chicken breast with skin side down and place over a medium flame and cook until skin is crisp.
4. Flip over and add cream to sage mixture and pour over duck. Cook until duck is done.
5. Add spinach to pot and cook until wilted.
6. Serve.

Servings: 1

**Nutrition Facts (per serving)**
Calories 798
Net Carbs 0g
Fats 71g
Protein 36 g
Fiber 1g

# Chicken Pot Pie

**Ingredients**

*For filling:*
Bacon (5 slices)
Garlic powder (1 teaspoon)
Cream cheese (8 oz.)
Spinach (6 cups)
Salt
Chicken thighs (6, boneless and skinless)
Onion powder (1 teaspoon)
Celery seed (3/4 teaspoon)
Cheddar cheese (4 oz.)
Chicken broth (1/4 cup)

*For crust:*
Psyllium Husk Powder (3 tablespoons)
Eggs (1)
Cheddar cheese (1/4 cup)
Garlic powder (1/4 teaspoon)
Salt
Almond flour (1/3 cup)
Butter (3 tablespoons)
Cream cheese (1/4 cup)
Paprika (1/2 teaspoon)
Onion powder (1/4 teaspoon)
Black pepper

**Directions**
1. Cube chicken and season with black pepper and salt.
2. Set oven to 375 °F.
3. Use spices to season chicken and place into an oven proof skillet and place onto fire and cook until golden on the outside. Add bacon to pan and cook until golden.
4. Add broth to pan along with cheeses and stir to combine. Put in spinach in pan and cook until wilted.

5. Combine dry ingredients for crust in a bowl and add cheddar and cream cheese to a microwave safe dish and then add cheese and combine. Add mixture to dry ingredients and mix together.
6. Form crust, stir ingredients in pot and top with crust and use fork to pierce crust all over.
7. Bake for 15 minutes, take from oven and cool.
8. Serve.

Servings: 8

**Nutrition Facts (per serving)**
Calories 434
Net Carbs 3.4g
Fats 35.6g
Protein 20.4 g
Fiber 3.6g

# Chicken Parmesan

**Ingredients**

*For Chicken:*
Chicken breasts (3)
Mozzarella cheese (1 cup)
Salt
Black pepper

*For coating:*
Flaxseed meal (1/4 cup)
Oregano (1 teaspoon)
Black pepper (1/2 teaspoon)
Garlic powder (1/2 teaspoon)
Egg (1)
Pork rinds (2.5 oz.)
Parmesan cheese (1/2 cup)
Salt (1/2 teaspoon)
Red pepper flakes (1/4 teaspoon)
Paprika (2 teaspoons)
Chicken broth (1 ½ teaspoons)

*For Sauce:*
Tomato sauce (1 cup, low carb)
Garlic (2 cloves)
Salt
Olive oil (1/2 cup)
Oregano (1/2 teaspoon)
Black pepper

**Directions**
1. Add flax meal, spices, pork rinds and parmesan cheese in a processor and grind until combined.
2. Pound chicken breast and whisk egg with broth in a container. Add all ingredients for sauce to a pan stir and put over a low flame to cook.
3. Dip chicken in egg and then coat with dry mixture.
4. Heat oil in a pan and fry chicken then transfer to a casserole dish. Top with sauce and mozzarella and bake for 10 minutes.

5. Serve.

Servings: 4

**Nutrition Facts (per serving)**
Calories 646
Net Carbs 4g
Fats 46.8g
Protein 49.3g
Fiber 2.8g

# Bell Peppers Stuffed Korean Beef

**Ingredients**

Ground beef (1 lb.)
Spring onions (2, sliced)
Ginger (2 teaspoons, diced)
Eggs (8)
Bell peppers (2, cut in half)
Garlic (2 teaspoons, diced)
Salt
Black pepper

For Sauce:
Rice wine vinegar (1 ½ tablespoons)
Chili paste (1 tablespoon)
Apricot preserves (1/3 cup, sugar free)
Ketchup (1 tablespoon, low sugar)
Soy sauce (1 tablespoon)

**Directions**

1. Season beef with pepper and salt and start cooking over a medium flame until browned. Add ginger and garlic and stir together.
2. Push beef to one side and put in spring onions, cook for 2 minutes then stir together with beef. Take from flame and put aside.
3. Add all sauce ingredients to a pan and cook for 3 minutes then add half to beef.
4. Stir sauce and beef together and use to stuff peppers.
5. Set oven to 350 F and bake for 15 minutes.
6. Top with reserved sauce and serve.

Servings: 4

**Nutrition Facts (per serving)**

Calories 470
Net Carbs 6.3g
Fats 35g
Protein 32.3g
Fiber 5.3g

# Creamy Tarragon Chicken

**Ingredients**
Chicken breast (5 oz.)
Onion (1/4, sliced)
Chicken broth (1/2 cup)
Grain mustard (1 teaspoon)
Salt
Olive oil (1 tablespoon)
Mushrooms (3 oz.)
Heavy cream (1/4 cup)
Tarragon (1/2 teaspoon, dried)
Black pepper

**Directions**
1. Cube chicken and season with pepper and salt.
2. Heat oil in a pan and sauté chicken for 6 minutes until golden all over. Take from pan and put aside.
3. Add mushrooms and cook for 3 minutes until golden then add onion and cook for 3 minutes until soft and translucent.
4. Add broth and bring to a boil for 4 minutes then add remaining ingredients and adjust black pepper and salt to taste.
5. Return chicken to sauce in pan and cook for 5 minutes.
6. Serve.

Servings: 1

**Nutrition Facts (per serving)**
Calories 490
Net Carbs 5g
Fats 40g
Protein 32 g
Fiber 1g

# Beanless Chili con Carne

**Ingredients**
Ground beef (1 lb.)
Green pepper (1, chopped)
Onion (1, chopped)
Curry powder (2 tablespoons)
Cumin (2 tablespoons)
Coconut oil (1 tablespoon)
Onion powder (1 teaspoon)
Black pepper (1 teaspoon)
Italian sausage (1 lb., spicy)
Yellow pepper (1, chopped)
Tomato sauce (16 oz.)
Chili powder (2 tablespoons)
Garlic (1 tablespoon, diced)
Butter (1 tablespoon)
Salt (1 teaspoon)

**Directions**
1. Heat oil and butter in a pan, heat thoroughly and add garlic, onions and bell peppers. Cook for 3 minutes then add beef and sausage.
2. Cook for 5 minutes until browned then add onion and chili powder. Stir to combine and add tomato sauce. Lower flame and cook for 20 minutes.
3. Add cumin and curry, stir and cook for 45 minutes or until chili thickens to your liking.
4. Serve.

Servings: 5

**Nutrition Facts (per serving)**
Calories 415
Net Carbs 6g
Fats 25g
Protein 146 g
Fiber 51g

# Seared Ribeye Steak

**Ingredients**
Ribeye steaks (2 medium)
Salt
Black pepper
Bacon fat (3 tablespoons)

**Directions**
1. Set oven to 250 ℉.
2. Place a wire rack over a baking sheet and place steaks on rack.
3. Use pepper and salt to season steaks and bake until steak's internal temperature is 123 ℉.
4. Melt fat in a cast iron pan until it is extremely hot then transfer steaks to pot and sear on both sides.
5. Let steaks sit for a few minutes before slicing.
6. Serve.

Servings: 5

**Nutrition Facts (per serving)**
Calories 430
Net Carbs 0g
Fats 31.7g
Protein 30.3 g

# Italian Fish Stew

### Ingredients
4 200g Kingklip fish fillets
2 onions, finely chopped
4 garlic cloves, minced
2 tins peeled, chopped tomato
4 tbsp. tomato paste
250ml white wine
½ tsp. parsley, chopped
¼ tsp. dried oregano
salt and pepper to taste
½ cup olive oil
1 cup water

### Directions
1. Preheat oven to 360C
2. Sauté onion and garlic on a pot then add tinned tomatoes and tomato paste and stir.
3. Pour the wine, parsley, oregano, salt, pepper, and water. Stir well and bring to a simmer.
4. Let it simmer for 10-15 minutes to reduce and thicken.
5. Meanwhile, place your fish in baking dish.
6. When sauce is nice and thick, pour it over fish and sprinkle with a little extra oregano.
7. Cover the dish with foil and place in the oven to cook for 20 minutes.
8. Take foil off and return to oven uncovered and cook for another 10 minutes.

**Tip:** If the sauce is a little runny when fish comes out, place sauce in another pot and put on heat to reduce a little more. Then pour back over fish.

**Nutrition Facts** (per serving)
Calories: 315
Net Carbs: 12
Fat: 8g
Protein: 37g

# Chicken Stir-Fry

**Ingredients**

4 chicken breasts (butterfly), marinate in egg white overnight
2 cups red pepper
2 cups mange tout
2 cups grated carrot
2 cups broccoli
2 cups almonds
2 cloves of garlic
½ tsp. ginger
2 tbsp. soya sauce
125ml chicken stock.
2 tbsp. coconut oil

**Directions**

1. Heat coconut oil in a pan over medium fire. Sauté the garlic and ginger until fragrant.
2. Cook the chicken breast in the oil and then add the vegetables. Toss and cook until almost done.
3. Add 2 tbsp. soya sauce and 125ml chicken stock. Allow to simmer uncovered until the broth evaporates.

**Nutrition Facts**

Calories: 186
Net Carbs: 4g
Fat: 11g
Protein: 17g

# Pan Fried Hake

**Ingredients**
1 tbsp. olive oil
Salt and pepper to taste
1 250g Hake fillet
fresh lemon wedges

**Directions**
1.  Heat the olive oil in a large frying pan over medium-high heat.
2.  Pat the fish dry with kitchen paper towel and then season with salt and pepper on both sides.
3.  Fry the fish for about 4-5 minutes on each side, depending on their thickness, or until they have a golden crust and the flesh flakes away easily with a fork.

**Nutrition Facts** (per serving)
Calories: 170
Net Carbs: 7g
Fat: 8g
Protein: 18g

# Creamed Spinach

**Ingredients**

2 cups spinach
½ small onion, chopped
¼ cup water
½ stock cube
1 clove of garlic, chopped
½ cup heavy cream
2 tbsp. butter
salt and pepper to taste

**Directions**

1. Place spinach and onion to a pan with water and heat over medium-high fire.
2. Add stock cube and garlic and allow to steam for 8-10 minutes or until all the water has evaporated and the spinach is very soft.
3. Pour in the heavy cream and butter and then season with salt and pepper. Cooking until it thickens.
4. Using a hand-held blender blitz the spinach until fairly smooth.
5. Serve while hot

**Nutrition Facts** (1/2 cup)

Calories: 200
Net Carbs: 3g
Fat: 23g
Protein: 7g

# Chicken and Mushroom Stew

**Ingredients**

8 pcs. chicken thighs
4 tbsp. butter
3 cloves garlic, minced
6 cups mushrooms
1 cup chicken stock
½ tsp. dried thyme
½ tsp. dried oregano
½ tsp. dried basil
¼ cup heavy cream
½ cup parmesan cheese, grated
1 tbsp. whole-grain mustard

**Directions**

1. Preheat oven to 400F
2. Season chicken thighs with salt and pepper
3. Heat an oven-proof pan over medium fire and melt 2 tbsp. of butter.
4. Add the chicken, skin-side down, and fry both sides until golden brown, or about 2-3 minutes per side. Set aside.
5. Melt remaining 2 tbsp. butter. Add garlic, thyme, oregano and basil and mushrooms, and cook, stirring occasionally. Cook until browned, about 5-6 minutes, season with salt and pepper, to taste.
6. Stir in chicken stock, then chicken back to the pan.
7. Pour everything into a baking dish with the chicken.
8. Place into oven and roast until completely cooked through for about 25-30 minutes. Set aside chicken.
9. Transfer sauces back into the original pan.
10. Stir in heavy cream, parmesan cheese and mustard. Bring to a boil; reduce heat and simmer until slightly reduced, about 5 minutes.
11. Serve chicken immediately, topped with mushroom mixture.

**Nutrition Facts** (1 serving)
Calories: 203
Net Carbs: 9g
Fat: 3g
Protein: 28g

# Beef Shin Stew

**Ingredients**

2 lb. quality shin of beef

4 tbsp. olive oil

2 red onions, peeled and roughly chopped

3 pcs. carrots, peeled and roughly chopped

3 sticks celery, trimmed and roughly chopped

4 cloves garlic, unpeeled

a few sprigs of fresh rosemary

2 bay leaves

2 cups mushrooms

2 cups baby marrows

salt and pepper to taste

1 tbsp. psyllium husk

2 cans 400 g tomatoes

⅔ bottle red wine

**Directions**

1. Preheat your oven to 360F
2. In a heavy-bottomed oven-proof saucepan, heat olive oil and sauté the onions, carrots, celery, garlic, herbs, and mushrooms for 5 minutes until softened slightly.
3. Meanwhile, toss the pieces of beef in the psyllium husk, shaking off any excess.
4. Add the meat to the pan and stir everything together.
5. Add the tomatoes, wine and a pinch of salt and pepper and gently bring to the boil.
6. Turn off heat then cover the sauce pan with a double-thickness piece of tinfoil and a lid and place in oven to cook for 3 hours or until the beef is meltingly tender and can be broken up with a spoon. Taste and check the seasoning remove the rosemary sprigs and serve hot.

**Nutrition Facts** (1 serving)

Calories: 315

Net Carbs: 7g

Fat: 7g

Protein: 20g

# Bacon, Beef Sausage and Broccoli Casserole

### Ingredients
500 g beef sausage
1/2 head of broccoli
8 slices of bacon
1/2 cup of cream
1 tbsp. Dijon mustard
100 g grated cheddar cheese

### Directions
1. Preheat oven to 350F
2. Slice the sausage and place in a small baking dish.
3. Slice the bacon and add to the sausage.
4. Break the broccoli into florets and arrange between the meat.
5. Mix the cream and mustard in a bowl and pour it all over the casserole, then top with the cheese.
6. Bake in the oven for 35 minutes.

### Nutrition Facts (1 serving)
Calories: 300
Net Carbs: 3g
Fat: 25g
Protein: 20g

# Creamy Haddock

**Ingredients**
150g smoked haddock
100ml boiling water
1 tbsp. butter
50ml cream
2 cups spinach

**Directions**
1. Heat a saucepan over medium fire.
2. Mix the boiling water with cream and butter in a bowl.
3. Place haddock and sauce in the pan and leave to boil until the water evaporates, leaving a creamy, butter sauce behind.
4. Serve haddock, covered with the sauce on fresh or wilted spinach.

**Nutrition Facts** (1 serving)
Calories: 281
Net Carbs: 15g
Fat: 10g
Protein: 18g

# Cauliflower Bake

**Ingredients**
4 slices of bacon
2 cups broccoli
2 cups cauliflower
2 cups mushrooms
1 green pepper
1 onion
200ml cream
120g cheese, grated
2 tbsp. olive oil

**Directions**
1. Preheat oven at 360F.
2. Steam or cook the cauliflower and broccoli until tender then transfer in an oven-proof dish.
3. Fry the bacon slices, with the mushrooms, green pepper and onion in 2 tbsp. olive oil.
4. Pour the fried bacon and mushrooms on top of cauliflower.
5. In a bowl, whisk 4 eggs with the cream and season to taste and pour over cauliflower or broccoli.
6. Place in the oven to cook for 25 minutes. Take out of the oven and sprinkle with grated cheese.
7. Place back in the oven and cook for another 5 minutes.

**Nutrition Facts** (1 serving)
Calories: 100
Net Carbs: 7g
Fat: 6g
Protein: 4g

# Caulicake

**Ingredients**

600 g cauliflower florets

1 onion, chopped

3 cloves of garlic, finely chopped

1 tsp. turmeric

100g parmesan cheese, finely grated

100g mature white cheddar cheese, coarsely grated

8 eggs

1-2 tsp. salt

2 tbsp. psyllium husk

1 cup of cream

1 tbsp. coconut oil

sesame seeds

olive oil

**Directions**

1. Preheat oven at 360F
2. Steam the cauliflower. Keep half of it whole and mash the rest.
3. Sauté the onion, garlic, turmeric in the coconut oil until soft. Set aside.
4. In a separate bowl, whisk the eggs. Add the cream, cheese, salt, and psyllium husk.
5. Combine the cauliflower, whole and mashed with the sautéed onions and egg mixture in a bowl.
6. Line a spring-form baking tin with greased baking paper and sprinkle with sesame seeds. Place the pan onto a baking tray.
7. Pour in the cauliflower mix and bake in the oven for 40 minutes.
8. As soon as it comes out of the oven, lightly prick the surface all over with a fork and drizzle with olive oil.

**Nutrition Facts** (1 serving)

Calories: 160

Net Carbs: 5g

Fat: 11g

Protein: 8g

# Burger Patties

**Ingredients**
500g ground beef
1 small onion, finely chopped
1 red pepper, chopped
¼ cup cheese, grated
1 carrot, grated
1 baby marrow, grated
1 tsp. ginger, grated
1 tsp. crushed garlic
2 eggs
2 tbsp. almond flour
1 tsp. parsley, minced
1 tsp. coriander
Salt and pepper to take

**Directions**
1. Mix all ingredients together in a bowl.
2. Form the mixture into balls and flatten into patties.
3. Roll the patties in almond flour and leave to firm in the fridge for around 30 minutes. This will help to keep the patties from falling apart while cooking.
4. When firm, pan fry the patties in coconut oil. Make sure your oil is hot before adding patties to the pan, you need to hear that oil sizzle. If the oil is not hot, the patty will stick to the pan and fall apart while cooking.
5. Take 1 large brown mushroom, rub with olive oil and some crushed garlic, do not salt. And bake in the oven at 360F for 15-20mins. Place the cooked burger on top of the mushroom, add grated cheese and melt in the oven for a couple of minutes.
6. Add 1 tbsp. mayo to finely diced red onion, lettuce and tomato and place on top of burger.

**Nutrition Facts** (1 serving)
Calories: 340
Net Carbs: 3g
Fat: 28g
Protein: 17g

# Slow Cooker Oxtail Stew

**Ingredients**

1.5kg of oxtail
1 Large pack grated cabbage
1 Large pack grated carrots
2 Large onions
1 Large Bunch of celery
1 Tin of tomatoes
2 Jelly Stock Cubes
2.5 litres of water
1Tblsp Crushed garlic
1 branch Rosemary
2 Bay Leaves

**Directions**

1. Place all ingredients into a slow cooker and cook on medium for 9 hours.
   Season with salt and pepper
2. Grate 60g cheddar cheese to finish (optional).

**Serves 10**

# Chicken Hash

**Ingredients**
1 Tbsp. olive oil
1/4 onion finely diced
1 cups broccoli
1 cup chicken stock
50g chicken breast cooked and finely diced
½ tsp. salt
¼ tsp. black pepper
¼ cup pumpkin

**Directions**
1. Add all ingredients to chicken stock, cover and cook approximately 20 minutes

# Tuna Fish Stew

**Ingredients**

1 tin tuna in water, drained
1 Tbsp. butter
¼ small onion, chopped finely
1 clove garlic, minced
1 teaspoon fresh ginger, grated
½ tin tomatoes, chopped finely
1 cup spinach, chopped finely
1 small carrot, grated
1 teaspoon curry powder 1 teaspoon turmeric
½ teaspoon cayenne pepper (optional)
Salt & pepper to taste

**Directions**

1. Fry onion, garlic and ginger in butter.
2. Add tomatoes once onions are soft.
3. Add spices and enough water to make a stew for the spinach, carrot and tuna fish. Cook at low heat for about 15 minutes.
4. Do not overcook spinach.
5. Steam 2 cups of cauliflower, mash and add 1 Tblsp of butter. Serve stew on top of the cauli-mash.

# Ratatouille

*Serves 4*

**Ingredients**
2 large brinjals
1 large onion
2 peppers (can be green, red, yellow)
2 tins of chopped tomatoes
1 packet baby marrows
1 punnet mushrooms
1 packet spinach
500ml chicken stock
Salt & pepper
2 cloves garlic (finely chopped or pressed)

**Directions**
1. Finely chop all the ingredients.
2. Add all the finely chopped veggies, garlic and onion to the stock and boil on medium until the water has reduced, and the veggies have formed a thick delicious stew.
3. Serve with 150g chunky cottage cheese, 30g cheddar or 6Tblsp Parmesan Cheese

# Easy Roast Tomato Sauce

*Serves 10*

**Ingredients**
10 tomatoes
Bunch of fresh basil
Garlic, bulb
Olive oil
Salt and pepper

**Directions**
1. Preheat oven to 190C,
2. Slice 10 tomatoes in half lengthways
3. Add a bunch of fresh basil.
4. Cut an entire bulb of garlic through the middle and place each half face up in the baking tray/dish
5. Immerse the tomatoes in olive oil and grind salt and pepper (Himalayan).
6. Roast in oven for about 1 hour and then turn the oven off for another 30 mins and leave to sit in the warm oven.
7. Remove the tomatoes and allow to cool,
8. do not mix, as you want to squeeze the flesh and pips out of the skin and discard the skin, squeeze the garlic from the cloves and throw away the casings.
9. Mash with a fork

**Note:** This makes THE best roast tomato sauce for pizza's meatballs or any other protein. Freeze in small Ziploc bags or plastic containers. You can add onion, red and yellow peppers and fresh chill for more robust flavour. Use a hand blender to blitz if you want a smoother sauce.

# Tender Pork & Bacon Cassoulet

### Ingredients
1 pack bacon, fried and then crumbled
Chopped onion (2 cups)
Dried thyme (1 teaspoon)
Dried rosemary (1/2 teaspoon)
3 garlic cloves, crushed
Salt (1/2 teaspoon)
Freshly ground black pepper (1/2 teaspoon)
2 cans diced tomatoes, drained
500g boneless pork loin roast, trimmed and cut into 2cm cubes
250g smoked sausage, cut into 1cm cubes
Finely shredded fresh Parmesan cheese (8 teaspoons)
Chopped fresh flat-leaf parsley (8 teaspoons)

### Directions
1. Fry bacon onion, thyme, rosemary, and garlic, then add salt, pepper, and tomatoes; bring to a boil.
2. Remove from heat.
3. Place all ingredients in the slow cooker, alternating the meat with the tomato sauce until finished. Cover and cook on low for 5 hours. Sprinkle with Parmesan cheese and parsley when cooked

Servings: 4

### Nutrition Facts (per serving)
Calories- 258
Carbs- 10.8g
Protein- 27g
Fats- 12.6g

# Lamb Cutlets with Garlic Sauce

*Serves 6*

**Ingredients**
4 lbs. lamb cutlets
1 small head of garlic, cloves peeled
2 Tbsp. apple cider vinegar
1/2 cup water
1/4 cup extra virgin olive oil
pinch salt and black ground pepper to taste

**Directions**
1. Crush the garlic cloves thoroughly in a mortar. In a bowl, add the vinegar and water and mix it well with the crushed garlic. Set aside.
2. In a large frying pan, pour the olive oil and fry the lamb cutlets until nicely brown.
3. Add the garlic mixture and let it cook gently for about 10 minutes.
4. Shake the frying pan to spread the garlic mixture evenly over the lamb.
5. Season with salt and black pepper to taste. Serve.

Cooking Times: 40 minutes

**Nutrition Facts (per serving)**
Carbs 0,16g
Calories 416, 68
Fat 28,76g
Fiber 0,01g
Sugar 0,05g
Protein 36,68g

# Tangy Shrimp Soup

*Serves 8*

## Ingredients
12 oz. fresh shrimp, peeled and deveined
1 cup zucchini (medium, sliced)
1 onion, chopped
2 cloves garlic, minced
1 Tbsp. ginger, minced
1 pinch crushed red pepper
2 quarts water
1 cup celery (chopped)
2 cups cauliflower florets
2 Tbsp. soy sauce
1/4 tsp. ground black pepper
2 tsp. olive oil

## Directions
1. In a large saucepan with over medium heat cook onion, garlic, ginger and crushed red pepper for 2 minutes.
2. Pour in water, cauliflower florets and celery and bring to a boil. Reduce heat, cover and simmer 5 minutes.
3. Stir in zucchini and shrimp, season with salt and pepper to taste; cover and cook 5 - 7 minutes.
4. Stir in soy sauce and pepper and serve.

Cooking Times
Total Time: 25 minutes

## Nutrition Facts (per serving)
Carbs 7,12g
Calories 107, 62
Fat 3,08g
Fiber 1,6g
Sugar 3,35g
Protein 12,08g

# Baked Herb Salmon Fillets

*Serves 6*

## Ingredients
2 lbs. salmon fillets
1/2 cup chopped fresh mushrooms
1/2 cup chopped green onions
4 oz. butter
4 Tbsp. coconut oil
1/2 cup tamari soy sauce
1 tsp. minced garlic
1/4 tsp. thyme
1/2 tsp. rosemary
1/4 tsp. tarragon
1/2 tsp. ground ginger
1/2 tsp. basil
1 tsp. oregano leaves

## Directions
1. Preheat oven to 350 degrees F. Line a large baking pan with foil.
2. Cut salmon filet in pieces. Put the salmon into the Ziploc bag with the tamari sauce, sesame oil and spices sauce mixture. Refrigerate the salmon and marinade it for 4 hours.
3. Put the salmon in a baking pan and bake fillets for 10-15 minutes.
4. Melt the butter. Add the chopped fresh mushrooms and green onion to it, and mix. Remove the salmon from the oven, and pour the butter mixture over the salmon fillets, making sure each fillet gets covered. Bake for about 10 minutes more. Serve immediately.

Inactive Time: 4 hours
Cooking Time: 35 minutes

## Nutrition Facts (per serving)
Carbs 2,77g
Calories 449
Fat 34,11g
Fiber 0,72g
Protein 33,19g

241

# Snack Recipes

# Bacon & Onion Bites

*Serves 12*
Serving Size: 1 cookie

### Ingredients
Almond flour (1 ½ cups)
Flax meal (1/3 cup)
Psyllium husk powder (1 tablespoon)
Onion powder (1 tablespoon)
1 large egg
4 slices bacon, cooked until crispy and crumbled
Sea salt (1/2 teaspoon)
Freshly ground pepper

### Directions
1. Place all of the dry ingredients into a bowl (almond flour, flax meal, psyllium husk powder, onion powder, salt and pepper) and mix until well combined.
2. If you don't have onion powder, you can use dried onion flakes and blend them until powdered. Also, make sure you don't use whole psyllium husks - blend the psyllium husks until powdered if needed.
3. Add the egg and mix well using your hands.
4. Add the crumbled bacon to the dough. Process well using your hands.  (Be sure to save the bacon fat from the cooking process for other uses - like some of the other fat bomb recipes in this book.)
5. Using your hand, create 12 equal balls and place them on a baking sheet lined with parchment paper.
6. Use a fork to press and flatten the dough.

### Nutrition Facts (per serving)
Calories: 109
Fat: 9

# Parmesan Crisps

*Serves 4*
Serving Size: 5 crisps

## Ingredients
Parmesan cheese (1 cup)
Coconut flour (4 tablespoons)
Rosemary, oregano or any herbs of choice, dried or fresh (1-2 teaspoons)

## Directions
1. Preheat the oven to 350 Fahrenheit. In a small bowl, mix the coconut flour and grated parmesan cheese. Don't use finely grated or powdery parmesan cheese like you find in a canister at the supermarket, as it won't work well in this recipe. Try to find finely grated parmesan in the deli section of your supermarket, or even better, grate your own!
2. You can add any herbs you like. Oregano and rosemary work wonderfully.
3. Scoop a teaspoon of the cheese mixture onto a baking tray lined with parchment paper leaving a small gap between each. Place in the oven and cook for 10-15 minutes or until golden brown, but be careful not to burn.
4. Remove from the oven and let the crisps cool down before you remove them from the baking tray.
5. Enjoy!

## Nutrition Facts (per serving)
Calories: 233
Fat: 14.5

# Mini Pizza Queens

*Serves 6*

### Ingredients
14 slices Italian sausages
8 pitted black olives
3/4 cup Cream cheese
2 Tbs fresh basil, chopped
2 Tbs pesto
salt and pepper to taste

### Directions
1. Dice pitted Kalamata olives and pepperoni into small pieces.
2. Mix together cream cheese, basil and pesto.
3. Add the olives and sausage slices into the cream cheese and mix again.
4. Form into balls and garnish with pepperoni, basil, and olive. Ready!!

Cooking Time: 10 minutes

### Nutrition Facts (per serving)
Carbs: 3,5g
Protein: 10,4g
Fat: 23,43g
Calories: 261

# Cheesy Bacon Balls

*Serves 24*

### Ingredients
8 strips cooked crispy bacon, crumbled
1 cup cream cheese, softened
1/2 cup butter
4 tsp. bacon fat
4 Tbsp. coconut oil
1/4 cup Splenda to taste

### Directions
1. In a microwave dish, combine all ingredients and melt slowly in the microwave until smooth. Set aside some crumbled bacon,
2. Pour into a dish or pan and place in the freezer until firm, about 30 minutes.
3. Before serving, remove from freezer, sprinkle with more crumbled bacon, slice and serve.

### Nutrition Facts (per serving)
Carbs: 0,5g
Fiber: 0g
Protein: 0g
Fat: 15,9g
Calories: 151

# Creamy Greek Balls

*Serves 5*

## Ingredients

1 cup cream cheese, softened
1 cup butter, softened
2-3 Tbsp. freshly chopped herbs (any combination of basil, thyme, oregano and/or parsley works great) or 2 teaspoons of dried herbs
4 pieces sun-dried tomatoes, drained
4 Kalamata olives, pitted and chopped
2 cloves garlic, crushed
freshly ground black pepper
1 tsp. sea salt
5 Tbs parmesan cheese, finely grated

## Directions

1. Mash the butter and cream cheese together with a fork and mix until well combined. Mix in the chopped sun-dried tomatoes and chopped Kalamata olives.
2. Add the freshly chopped herbs (or dried), crushed garlic and season with salt and pepper. Mix well and place in the fridge for 20-30 minutes to firm up.
3. Remove the cheese mixture from the fridge and start creating 5 balls. A spoon or an ice-cream scooper works well.
4. Place the grated parmesan cheese in a shallow dish. Roll each ball in the grated parmesan cheese and place on a plate. Eat immediately or store in the fridge in an airtight container for up to a week.
5. Enjoy!

## Nutrition Facts (per serving)

Carbs: 2,8g
Fiber: 0,24g
Protein: 3,67g
Fat: 19,8g
Calories: 200

# Smoked Turkey, Blue Cheese Eggs

*Serves 6*

**Ingredients**
6 eggs
2 green onions
6 oz. smoked turkey breast, chopped
1/2 cup blue cheese, crumbled
2 Tbsp. Blue cheese dressing
1/4 cup mayonnaise
2 Tbsp. hot mustard
1/2 rib celery

**Directions**
1. Hard boil the eggs, covered for 12 minutes.
2. In a meanwhile, chop up the smoked turkey breast and the celery.
3. Slice eggs in half lengthwise, scrape the yolks out into a bowl. Add the rest of the ingredients (except the green onions).
4. Grate the green onions over the mixture. Mix all ingredients together.
5. With the teaspoon fill every egg with the mixture.
6. Place on a serving plate and refrigerate for one hour. Ready! Serve and enjoy!

Cooking Times
Total Time: 20 minutes

**Nutrition Facts (per serving)**
Carbs: 3,9g
Fiber: 0,3g
Protein: 14g
Fat: 11,5g
Calories: 167

# Pancetta & Eggs

*Serves 4*

**Ingredients**
4 large slices Pancetta
2 eggs, free-range
1 cup ghee, softened
2 Tbsp. mayonnaise
salt and freshly ground black pepper to taste
coconut oil for frying

**Directions**
1. In a greased non-stick frying pan, bake Pancetta from both sides 1-2 minutes. Remove from the fire and set aside.
2. In a meanwhile boil the eggs. To get the eggs hard-boiled, you need round 10 minutes. When done, wash the eggs with cold water well and peel off the shells.
3. In a deep bowl place ghee and add the quartered eggs. Mash with a fork well. Season it with salt and pepper to taste; add mayonnaise and mix. If you want you can pour in the Pancetta grease. Combine and mix well. Place the bowl in the fridge for one hour at least.
4. Remove the egg mixture from the fridge and make 4 equal balls.
5. Crumble the Pancetta into small pieces. Roll each ball in the Pancetta crumbles and place on a big platter.
6. Remove the Egg and Pancetta bombs in a fridge for 30 minutes more. Serve cold.

**Nutrition Facts (per serving)**
Carbs: 2,2g
Fiber: 0g
Protein: 7,5g
Fat: 22g
Calories: 238

# Parmesan, Herb & Sun-dried Tomato Bombs

*Serves 4*

**Ingredients**
1 cup cream cheese
1 cup ghee
5 Tbsp. parmesan cheese
1/4 cup sun-dried tomatoes, chopped
1/4 cup Kalamata olives, pitted
3 cloves garlic, crushed
3 Tbsp. herbs mix (basil, parsley, thyme, oregano, parsnip, mint)
salt and freshly ground black pepper to taste

**Directions**
1. In a bowl, combine the cream cheese and ghee. Set aside for 30-45 minutes to soft.
2. After, mix the ghee and the cream cheese until well combined. Add the chopped Kalamata olives and sun-dried tomatoes.
3. Add in herbs and crushed garlic; season with salt and pepper to taste. Mix well with the fork and place bowl in the fridge for at least 1 hour.
4. Remove the cheese mixture from the fridge and create 4 balls. Roll each ball in the grated parmesan cheese and place on a plate.
5. Return it to the fridge for 30 minutes. Serve and enjoy.

Cooking Times
Total Time: 1 hour and 20 minutes

**Nutrition Facts (per serving)**
Carbs: 4g
Fiber: 0,5g
Protein: 4,6g
Fat: 14g
Calories: 157

# Spicy Bacon & Avo Bites

*Serves 6*
*Serving Size: 1 bite*

## Ingredients
½ large avocado
Butter, softened (1/4 cups)
2 cloves garlic, crushed
Crushed red pepper (1 teaspoon)
½ small white onion, diced
Fresh lime juice (1 tablespoon)
Freshly ground black pepper
Sea salt (¼ teaspoon)
large slices bacon
Bacon grease, reserved from cooking (2 tablespoons)

## Directions
1. Preheat the oven to 375 Fahrenheit. Line a baking tray with parchment paper. Lay the bacon strips out flat on the parchment paper, leaving space so they don't overlap. Place the tray in the oven and cook for about 10-15 minutes until golden brown and crisp. The time will depend on the thickness of the bacon slices. When done, remove from the oven and set aside to cool down.
2. Halve, deseed and peel the avocado. Place the avocado, butter, crushed red pepper, crushed garlic and lime juice into a bowl and season with salt and pepper.
3. Mash using a potato masher or a fork until well combined. Add the diced onion and mix well.
4. Pour in the 2 tablespoons of reserved bacon grease and mix well. Cover with foil and place in the fridge for 20-30 minutes to firm up.
5. Chop the bacon into small pieces and place in a shallow dish.
6. Remove the guacamole mixture from the fridge and start creating 6 balls. You can use a spoon or an ice-cream scooper. Roll each ball in the bacon crumbles and place on a tray that will fit in the fridge.
7. Eat immediately or store in the fridge in an airtight container for up to 5 days.

## Nutrition Facts (per serving)
Calories: 156
Fat: 15.2

# Fried Tuna & Avo Balls

*Serves 12*

**Ingredients**
Mayonnaise (1/4 cup)
Parmesan cheese (1/4 cup)
Garlic powder (1/2 teaspoon)
Salt
Canned Tuna (10 oz., drained)
Avocado (1, cubed)
Almond flour (1/3 cup)
Onion powder (1/4 teaspoon)
Coconut oil (1/2 cup)

**Directions**
1. Combine all ingredients in a bowl except oil and avocado.
2. Add avocado and fold, use hands to form balls and dust with flour.
3. Heat oil in a pot and fry tuna bites until golden all over.
4. Serve.

**Nutrition Facts (per serving) per bite**
Calories 135
Net Carbs 0.8g
Fats 11.8g
Protein 6.2 g
Fiber 1.2g

# Bacon Zucchini Fat Bomb Balls

**Ingredients**

1 lbs. smoked bacon, crumbled
1 cup pork rinds, crushed
5 cups zucchini, minced
4 cloves garlic, minced
1 cup cream cheese
2 1/2 cup grated Parmesan cheese
4 oz. goat cheese
1 tsp. onion powder
1 tsp. garlic powder
salt and freshly ground black pepper to taste

**Directions**

1. Chop or blend zucchini.
2. In large mixing bowl, combine bacon, zucchini, cream cheese, goat cheese, 1 cup grated Parmesan, minced garlic, salt and pepper to taste.  Mix until all ingredients are well incorporated.  Refrigerate for 2- 3 hours.
3. In a meanwhile prepare breading; in a bowl, combine crushed pork rinds, remaining 1 cup Parmesan cheese, onion powder and garlic powder.
4. Remove the zucchini mixture from the fridge and prepare about 30 even balls.
5. Roll each ball in Parmesan breading mixture until well and evenly coated. In a frying pan heat the oil.
6. Fry the zucchini bolls until they are a nice even golden brown all over. Place on a serving plate and serve hot.

Servings: 30
Cooking Time: 20 minutes

**Nutrition Facts (per serving)**
Carbs: 1,7g
Fiber: 0,25g
Protein: 7g
Fat: 13g
Calories: 151

# Baked Creamy Shrimps with Artichoke Hearts

**Ingredients**
6 oz. shrimp, precooked
2 Tbsp. butter
1 can (11 oz.) artichoke hearts, chopped
6 scallions
1/2 cup mayonnaise
1/2 cup sour cream
1 cup Cheddar cheese, shredded
1 1/4 cup Parmesan cheese, shredded
1 Tbsp. garlic, minced
1 tsp. red pepper flakes
1 tsp. garlic powder

**Directions**
1. Preheat oven to 350F.
2. In a frying pan, sauté shrimps over medium heat with butter and red pepper flakes for 5-10 minutes. Chop the artichoke hearts.
3. In a bowl, combine all your ingredient and mix until well blended.
4. Pour the mixture in a baking dish and bake for 30 minutes in preheated oven. Serve hot.

Servings: 16
Cooking Times
Total Time: 40 minutes

**Nutrition Facts (per serving)**
Carbs: 6,32g
Fiber: 1,6g
Protein: 8g
Fat: 11g
Calories: 150

# Blue Cheese Turkey Dressed Eggs

**Ingredients**

6 eggs
2 green onions
6 oz. smoked turkey breast, chopped
1/2 cup blue cheese, crumbled
2 Tbsp. Blue cheese dressing
1/4 cup mayonnaise
2 Tbsp. hot mustard
1/2 rib celery

**Directions**

1. Hard boil the eggs, covered for 12 minutes.
2. In a meanwhile, chop up the smoked turkey breast and the celery.
3. Slice eggs in half lengthwise, scrape the yolks out into a bowl. Add the rest of the ingredients (except the green onions).
4. Grate the green onions over the mixture. Mix all ingredients together.
5. With the teaspoon fill every egg with the mixture.
6. Place on a serving plate and refrigerate for one hour. Ready! Serve and enjoy!

Servings: 6

Cooking Times
Total Time: 20 minutes

**Nutrition Facts (per serving)**

Carbs: 3,9g
Fiber: 0,3g
Protein: 14g
Fat: 11,5g
Calories: 167

# Olives and Sun-dried Tomatoes Fat Bombs

**Ingredients**

1 cup cream cheese

1 cup ghee

5 Tbsp. parmesan cheese

1/4 cup sun-dried tomatoes, chopped

1/4 cup Kalamata olives, pitted

3 cloves garlic, crushed

3 Tbsp. herbs mix (basil, parsley, thyme, oregano, parsnip, mint)

salt and freshly ground black pepper to taste

**Directions**

1. In a bowl, combine the cream cheese and ghee. Set aside for 30-45 minutes to soft.
2. After, mix the ghee and the cream cheese until well combined. Add the chopped Kalamata olives and sun-dried tomatoes.
3. Add in herbs and crushed garlic; season with salt and pepper to taste. Mix well with the fork and place bowl in the fridge for at least 1 hour.
4. Remove the cheese mixture from the fridge and create 4 balls. Roll each ball in the grated parmesan cheese and place on a plate.
5. Return it to the fridge for 30 minutes. Serve and enjoy.

Servings: 4

Cooking Times

Total Time: 1 hour and 20 minutes

**Nutrition Facts (per serving)**

Carbs: 4g

Fiber: 0,5g

Protein: 4,6g

Fat: 14g

Calories: 157

# Pork Ham, Sausages and Cashews Truffles

**Ingredients**

8 slices smoked pork ham

8 oz. sausages

6 oz. cream cheese, softened

1 cup cashews, chopped

1 tsp. Dijon mustard

**Directions**

1. In a food processor blend chopped sausages and cashews.
2. In a separate bowl, beat the cream cheese and mustard until soft.
3. Roll the sausage mixture into 12 small balls. Take each ball and form layer of cream cheese with your fingers.
4. Refrigerate for about 45-60 minutes.
5. Roll each ball in the finely chopped smoked pork ham and place on a serving dish. Serve.

Servings: 12

Total Time: 15 minutes

**Nutrition Facts (per serving)**

Carbs: 1,5g

Protein: 7g

Fat: 11g

Calories: 125

# Smoked Mackerel Bombs

### Ingredients
2 oz. smoked mackerel fish
2.7 oz. butter, grass-fed
3.5 oz. cream cheese
1 Tbsp. fresh lemon juice
pinch of salt

### Directions
1. In a food processor put butter, cream cheese, smoked mackerel fish and fresh lemon juice. Blend until all ingredients incorporate well.
2. Line a tray with parchment paper and create 6 fat bombs. Place in the fridge for 2 hours or until firm. Serve.

Servings: 6
Cooking Time: 5 minutes

### Nutrition Facts (per serving)
Carbs: 0,8g
Protein: 3,3g
Fat: 17g
Calories: 163

# Bacon Bomb Dip

**Ingredients**

6 slices bacon, cooked and crumbled

2 cups sour cream

1 cup cream cheese

1 1 cups Cheddar cheese, shredded

1 cup sliced scallions, white and green parts

**Directions**

1. Preheat oven to 400 F
2. In a deep bowl, combine all ingredients. Spoon mixture into a baking dish and bake until cheese is bubbling, about 25-30 minutes.
3. Once ready, let cool and serve hot.

Servings: 18

Cooking Time: 35 minutes

**Nutrition Facts (per serving)**

Carbs: 1,7g

Protein: 5,5g

Fat: 19g

Calories: 197

# Turkey Bacon and Avocado Stuffed Eggs

**Ingredients**

6 eggs
1 avocado
6 slices smoked turkey bacon
2 Tbsp. mustard
1 Tbsp. garlic, minced
1 Tbsp. lime juice
1 Tbsp. dried onion flakes
pinch Cayenne pepper, or to taste
1 tsp. garlic salt

**Directions**

1. Hard boil the eggs (about 12 minutes). Peel the eggs and slice in half lengthwise
2. In a large mixing bowl mash the avocado.
3. Scrape the yolks out into the mixing bowl. Add in the bacon, mustard, cayenne pepper, lime juice, onion flakes, garlic and garlic salt. Mix it well until smooth and creamy.
4. Fill every egg half with the avocado mixture. Refrigerate stuffed eggs for one hour. Serve.

Servings: 6

Cooking Times
Total Time: 30 minutes

**Nutrition Facts (per serving)**
Carbs: 4,4g
Fiber: 2,3g
Protein: 9g
Fat: 13g
Calories: 162
Protein 9,36g

# Hot Pepperoni Bombs

**Ingredients**
1/2 cup Cream cheese
4 slices  Pepperoni Sausages (or any salami made from cured pork and beef mixed together)
3 slices smoked bacon
1 medium Chili pepper
1/2 tsp. dried basil
1/4 tsp. onion powder
1/4 tsp. garlic powder
salt and pepper to taste

**Directions**
1. In a frying pan brown 3 slices of bacon  and Peperoni sausages until crisp.
2. Remove bacon and Pepperoni from the pan on a paper lined plate to cool. Keep the remaining grease for later use.
3. Dice Chilli pepper into small pieces.
4. Combine cream cheese, chilli pepper and spices.  Add the bacon fat in and mix together until a solid mixture is formed. Season with salt and pepper to taste.
5. Crumble bacon and Pepperone slices and set on a plate. Roll cream cheese mixture into balls using your hand, then roll the ball into the bacon or Pepperone.

Servings: 6

**Cooking Times**
Total Time: 15 minutes

**Nutrition Facts (per serving)**
Carbs: 1,3g
Fiber: 0,11g
Protein: 4g
Fat: 16g
Calories: 165

# Wrapped Bacon Rolls

### Ingredients
4 bacon slice
6 toasted pecan halves, chopped
1/2 cup unsalted butter
1/2 cup of Mayonnaise
granulated garlic (to taste)

### Directions
1. Divide bacon into 3 equal parts.
2. Spread generously each bacon part with unsalted butter. Press butter side into pecan pieces.
3. Top with each with a mayonnaise, sprinkle with granulated garlic and wrap in a rolls. Enjoy!!

Servings: 12

Cooking Time: 10 minutes

### Nutrition Facts (per serving)
Carbs: 2,7g
Fiber: 0,15g
Protein: 1,78g
Fat: 17,7g
Calories: 174

# Lettuce with Prosciutto and Butternut Squash

**Ingredients**
3 strips Prosciutto
1 cup butternut squash, cubed
1/4 cup sour cream
3 Tbsp. thinly sliced fresh chives
6 lettuce leaves
Kosher salt and freshly ground black pepper

**Directions**
1.  In a frying pan, cook the bacon about 3 minutes. Add the butternut squash and salt and pepper to taste. Cook, stirring 6 - 8 minutes. Add in the chives and adjust salt and pepper to taste. Let cool for several minutes.
2.  Chop the bacon and add all other ingredients (except lettuce) and mix well.
3.  Set the lettuce leaves on a large platter. Top each leave with a dollop of the bacon-sour cream-butternut squash mixture and then sprinkle with some chopped chives. Serve immediately.

Servings: 6
Cooking Time: 35 minutes

**Nutrition Facts (per serving)**
Carbs: 4g
Protein: 2,76g
Fat: 11g
Calories: 120

# Pancetta Wrapped Provolone Sticks

### Ingredients
4 slices Pancetta bacon
2 Frigo string Provolone cheese (or Mozzarela, Kasseri, Emmenthal...)
1/2 cup coconut oil for frying
toothpicks

### Directions
1. Preheat your coconut oil in a deep fryer to 350 degrees.
2. Wrap your cut in half Provolone cheese sticks with the Pancetta. At the end of the wrapping, secure with a toothpick.
3. Drop the bacon wrapped cheese in the hot oil and cook about 2-3 minutes, depending on the thickness of your bacon.
4. Remove your Pancetta Wrapped Provolone Sticks to a paper towel to cool for a few minutes. Remove the toothpick and serve.

**Servings:** 10

### Nutrition Facts (per serving)
Carbs: 0,42g
Fiber: 0g
Protein: 5,6g
Fat: 22g
Calories: 216

# Savory Coco Bacon Bombs

**Ingredients**

8 strips cooked crispy bacon, crumbled

1 cup cream cheese, softened

1/2 cup butter

4 tsp. bacon fat

4 Tbsp. coconut oil

1/4 cup Splenda to taste

**Directions**

1. In a microwave dish, combine all ingredients and melt slowly in the microwave until smooth. Set aside some crumbled bacon,
2. Pour into a dish or pan and place in the freezer until firm, about 30 minutes.
3. Before serving, remove from freezer, sprinkle with more crumbled bacon, slice and serve.

**Servings: 24**

**Nutrition Facts (per serving)**

Carbs: 0,5g

Fiber: 0g

Protein: 0g

Fat: 15,9g

Calories: 151

# Scrambled Eggs Muffins

## Ingredients
3 strips of crumbled cooked bacon
6 six eggs
2 Tbsp. Coconut oil or butter
1 Tbsp. butter
1/4 cup softened cream cheese
1/4 cup shredded Gouda cheese
garlic & onion powder
black or white pepper

## Directions
1. In small bowl, melt the butter and set aside. In a separate bowl beat the eggs. Add in spices.Heat some butter in a non stick skillet on medium heat and scramble the eggs .
2. Put cooked eggs into another large bowl. Put in your cheeses and mix well. Add bacon and stir. Add the melted butter and coconut oil.
3. Pour the batter in mini muffin liners. Place on cookie sheet with or without wax paper, and freeze for about 30 minutes. Serve.

**Servings:** 8

**Cooking Times**
Total Time: 15 minutes

**Nutrition Facts (per serving)**
Carbs: 0,54g
Fiber: 0g
Protein: 7,9g
Fat: 16,9g
Calories: 186
Sugar 0,31g

# Smoked Salmon Cream Cheese Balls

**Ingredients**
2 oz smoked salmon fillets
1/2 cup cream cheese
3 oz butter, grass-fed
1 Tbs fresh lemon juice
pinch salt

**Directions**
1. In a food processor put butter, cream cheese, smoked mackerel and fresh lemon juice. Blend until all ingredients incorporate well.
2. Line a tray with parchment paper and create 6 Balls. Place in the fridge for 2 hours or until firm.
3. Serve.

**Servings**: 6
Cooking Time: 5 minutes

**Nutrition Facts (per serving)**
Carbs: 0,87g
Fiber: 0.1g
Protein: 3,29g
Fat: 16,62g
Calories: 163

# Breading Kohlrabi & Bacon Rind

**Ingredients**
1 lb smoked bacon, crumbled
5 cups kohlrabi, minced
1 cup pork rinds, crushed
2 1/2 cup grated Parmesan cheese
4 oz mascarpone cheese
4 cloves garlic, minced
1 cup cream cheese
1 tsp. onion powder
1 tsp. garlic powder
salt ad freshly ground black pepper to taste

**Directions**
1. Chop or blend kohlrabi.
2. In large mixing bowl, combine kohlrabi, bacon, cream cheese, mascarpone cheese, 1 cup grated Parmesan, minced garlic, salt and pepper to taste. Mix until all ingredients are well incorporated. Refrigerate for 2- 3 hours.
3. For breading: In a bowl, combine crushed pork rinds, remaining 1 cup Parmesan cheese, onion powder and garlic powder.
4. Remove the kohlrabi mixture from the fridge and prepare about 30 even balls.
5. In a frying pan heat the oil. Roll each ball in Parmesan breading mixture until well and evenly coated. Fry the kohlrabi balls until they are a nice even golden brown all over. Place on a serving plate and serve hot.

**Servings**: 30
**Cooking Times**
Total Time: 20 minutes

**Nutrition Facts (per serving)**
Carbs: 2,5g
Fiber: 0,9g
Protein: 7,5g
Fat: 13g
Calories: 154

# Dessert Recipe

# Chocolate Minty Ice Cream

*Serves 3*

**Ingredients**
1/2 tsp. Peppermint extract
1 cup heavy cream
1 cup cheese cream
1 tsp. pure vanilla extract
1 tsp. Liquid Stevia extract
100% Dark Chocolate for topping

**Directions**
1. Place ice cream bowl in freezer per ice cream maker instructions. In a metal bowl, put all ingredients except chocolate and whisk well.
2. Put back in freezer for 5 minutes. Setup ice cream maker and add liquid.
3. Before serving, top the ice cream with chocolate shavings. Serve.

Cooking Time: 35 minutes

**Nutrition Facts (per serving)**
Carbs 2,7g
Calories 286
Fat 29,96g
Sugar 0,9g
Protein 2,6g

# Coconut Waffles

*Serves 8*

## Ingredients
1 cup coconut flour
1/2 cup heavy (whipping) cream
5 eggs
1/4 tsp. pink salt
1/4 tsp. baking soda
1/4 cup coconut milk
2 tsp. Yacon Syrup (or some other natural sweetener)
2 Tbsp. coconut oil (melted)

## Directions
1. In a large bowl add the eggs and beat with an electric hand mixer for 30 seconds.
2. Add the heavy (whipping) cream and coconut oil into the eggs while you are still mixing. Add the coconut milk, coconut flour, pink salt and baking soda. Mix with the hand mixer for 45 second on low speed. Set aside.
3. Heat up your waffle maker well and make the waffles according to your manufactures specifications.
4. Serve hot.

## Nutrition Facts (per serving)
Calories 169
Fat 12,6g
Carbs 9,97g
Fiber 0,45g
Sugar 0,38g
Protein 4,39g

# Choc- Raspberry Cream

*Serves 4*

## Ingredients
1/2 cup 100% dark chocolate, chopped
1/4 cup of heavy cream
1/2 cup cream cheese, softened
2 Tbsp. sugar free Raspberry Syrup
1/4 cup Erythritol

## Directions
1. In a double boiler melt chopped chocolate and the cream cheese. Add the Erythritol sweetener and continue to stir. Remove from heat, let cool and set aside.
2. When the cream has cooled add in heavy cream and Raspberry syrup and stir well.
3. Pour cream in a bowls or glasses and serve. Keep refrigerated.

Cooking Time: 15 minutes

## Nutrition Facts (per serving)
Carbs 7,47g
Calories 157
Fat 13,51g
Fiber 1g
Sugar 5,16g
Protein 1,95g

# Hazelnut & Cacao Cookies

*Serves 24*

**Ingredients**
2 cups almond flour
1 cup chopped hazelnut
1/2 cup cacao powder
1/2 cup ground flax
3 Tbsp. coconut oil (melted)
1/3 cup water
1/3 cup Erythritol
1/4 tsp. liquid Stevia

**Directions**
1. In a bowl, mix almond flour and flax and cacao powder. Stir in oil, water, agave and vanilla. When it is well mixed, stir in chopped hazelnuts.
2. Form in to balls, press flat with palms and place on dehydrator screens.
3. Dehydrate 1 hour at 145, then reduce to 116 and dehydrate for at least 5 hours or until desired dryness is achieved.
4. Serve.

Cooking Time: 6 hours

**Nutrition Facts (per serving)**
Carbs 8,75g
Calories 181
Fat 15,69g
Fiber 3,45g
Sugar 3,75g
Protein 4,46g

# Dark Chocolate Brownies

*Serves 16*

### Ingredients
3 eggs
4 oz. dark chocolate, unsweetened
1/2 cup coconut oil
1 cup almond flour
1 cup walnuts
2 Tbsp. cocoa, unsweetened
1 tsp. vanilla essence
2 cups granulated sweetener Stevia or Erythritol
1 tsp. baking soda
pinch of salt

### Directions
1. Preheat the oven to 350F.
2. In a container, add almond flour, sweetener, cocoa, salt and baking soda. With an electric mixer, blend the ingredients on the slowest setting until combined well.
3. Melt the chocolate and the coconut oil together (In a microwave or double boiler). Stir thoroughly.
4. Add eggs and vanilla essence to the flour and mix on a medium speed until a thick batter is formed.
5. Add the butter/chocolate mix to the batter continuing on medium speed until an even texture is formed. Line a slice tin or square baking tin with wax paper. Fold in walnut pieces then turn the batter into your slice tin.
6. Bake for 25 minutes. When ready let cool on wire rack.
7. Cut into 16 Brownies and serve.

Cooking Time: 35 minutes

### Nutrition Facts (per serving)
Carbs 5,38g
Calories 207
Fat 20,72g
Fiber 2,82g
Sugar 0,73g
Protein 5,14g

# Rich Almond Butter Cake & Chocolate Sauce

*Serves 12*

## Ingredients
1 cup almond butter or soaked almonds
1/4 cup almond milk, unsweetened
1 cup coconut oil
2 tsp. liquid Stevia sweetener to taste

Topping: Chocolate Sauce
4 Tbsp. cocoa powder, unsweetened
2 Tbsp. almond butter
2 Tbsp. Stevia sweetener

## Directions
1. Melt the coconut oil in room temperature.
2. Add all ingredients in a bowl and blend well until combined.
3. Pour the almond butter mixture into a parchment lined platter.
4. Place in refrigerator for 3 hours.
5. In a bowl, whisk all topping ingredients together. Pour over the almond cake after it's been set. Cut into cubes and serve.

Cooking Time: 5 minutes

## Nutrition Facts (per serving)
Carbs: 9,8g
Fiber: 2g
Protein: 5,8g
Fat: 23,3g
Calories: 273

# Peanut Butter Cake Covered in Chocolate Sauce

*Serves 12*

**Ingredients**
1 cup peanut butter
1/4 cup almond milk, unsweetened
1 cup coconut oil
2 tsp. liquid Stevia sweetener to taste
Topping: Chocolate Sauce
2 Tbsp. coconut oil, melted
4 Tbsp. cocoa powder, unsweetened
2 Tbsp. Stevia sweetener

**Directions**
1.  In a microwave bowl mix coconut oil and peanut butter; melt in a microwave for 1-2 minutes.
2.  Add this mixture to your blender; add in the rest of the ingredients and blend well until combined.
3.  Pour the peanut mixture into a parchment lined loaf pan or platter.
4.  Refrigerate for about 3 hours; the longer, the better.
5.  In a bowl, whisk all topping ingredients together. Pour over the peanut candy after it's been set. Cut into cubes and serve.

Cooking Time: 5 minutes

**Nutrition Facts (per serving)**
Carbs: 5,8g
Fiber: 2g
Protein: 6g
Fat: 27g
Calories: 273

# Spicy Pumpkin Ice Cream

*Serves 6*

**Ingredients**
1 cup almond milk (unsweetened)
1 cup coconut milk
1 cup pumpkin puree
2 1/2 tsp. ground cinnamon
1 tsp. pure vanilla extract
1/2 tsp. ground ginger
1/2 tsp. nutmeg
1/8 tsp. sea salt
Thickener:
1/2 tsp. guar gum or 1 tablespoon gelatin dissolved in 1/4 cup boiling water

**Directions**
1. Put the coconut milk in a blender and purée until smooth.
2. Pour into the ice cream machine or blender and churn well. Serve in chilled glasses.
3. Freeze for about an hour or refrigerate until cold.
4. Add the almond milk, pumpkin puree, vanilla, cinnamon, ginger, nutmeg and salt, plus thickener. Purée until smooth.
5. Serve.

Cooking Times
Inactive Time: 1 hour
Total Time: 15 minutes

**Nutrition Facts (per serving)**
Carbs 4,73g
Calories 118
Fat 11,3g
Fiber 1,4g
Sugar 1,43g
Protein 1,35g

# All-stars Peanut-Butter Cookies

**Ingredients**
2 cups peanut butter
1/4 cup Erythritol
2 eggs
1 1/4 cups coconut flour
2 tsp. baking soda
2 tsp. peanut extract
1/2 tsp. kosher salt

**Directions**
1. Preheat oven to 345° F.
2. In a bowl beat the peanut butter, coconut flour and Erythritol with an electric mixer (MEDIUM speed) until fluffy. Reduce speed to LOW and add in the eggs, baking soda, vanilla, and salt.
3. With your hands make balls from the batter and place on parchment-lined baking pan. Bake 10 to 15 minutes. When ready, cool slightly and then move from the stove to cool completely. Ready. Serve.

Servings: 18

**Cooking Times**
Total Time: 1 hour and 15 minutes

**Nutrition Facts (per serving)**
Calories 182
Fat 14,67g
Carbs 8,65g
Fiber 1,96g
Protein 7g

# Pecan Blondie's

*Serves 16*

**Ingredients**
3 eggs
2 1/4 cups pecans, roasted
3 Tbsp. heavy cream
1 Tbsp. salted caramel syrup
1/2 cup flax seeds, ground
1/4 cup butter, melted
1/4 cup erythritol, powdered
10 drops Liquid Stevia
1 tsp. baking powder
1 pinch salt

**Directions**
1. Preheat oven to 350F.
2. In a baking pan roast pecans for 10 minutes.
3. Grind 1/2 cup flax seeds in a spice grinder. Place flax seed powder in a bowl. Grind Erythritol in a spice grinder until powdered. Set in the same bowl as the flax seeds meal.
4. Place 2/3 of roasted pecans in food processor and process until a smooth nut butter is formed.
5. Add eggs, liquid Stevia, salted caramel syrup, and a pinch of salt to the flax seed mixture. Mix well. Add pecan butter to the batter and mix again.
6. Smash the rest of the roasted pecans into chunks. Add crushed pecans and 1/4 cup melted butter into the batter.
7. Mix batter well, and then add heavy cream and baking powder. Mix everything together well.
8. Place the batter into baking tray and bake for 20 minute. Let cool for about 10 minutes. Slice off the edges of the brownie to create a uniform square. Serve.

Cooking Time: 40 minutes

**Nutrition Facts (per serving)**
Carbs 3,54g

Calories 180
Fat 18,23g
Fiber 1,78g
Sugar 1,45g
Protein 3,07g

# Chocolate Almond Brownies

**Ingredients**

3 eggs
4 oz. dark chocolate, unsweetened
1/2 cup coconut oil
1 cup almond flour
1 cup walnuts
2 Tbsp. cocoa, unsweetened
1 tsp. vanilla essence
2 cups granulated sweetener Stevia or Erythritol
1 tsp. baking soda
pinch of salt

**Directions**

1. Preheat the oven to 350F.
2. In a container, add almond flour, sweetener, cocoa, salt and baking soda. With an electric mixer, blend the ingredients on the slowest setting until combined well.
3. Melt the chocolate and the coconut oil together (In a microwave or double boiler). Stir thoroughly.
4. Add eggs and vanilla essence to the flour and mix on a medium speed until a thick batter is formed.
5. Add the butter/chocolate mix to the batter continuing on medium speed until an even texture is formed. Line a slice tin or square baking tin with wax paper. Fold in walnut pieces then turn the batter into your slice tin.
6. Bake for 25 minutes. When ready let cool on wire rack.
7. Cut into 16 Brownies and serve.

Servings: 16
**Cooking Times**: 35 minutes

**Nutrition Facts (per serving)**
Calories 207
Fat 20,72g
Carbs 5,38g
Fiber 2,82g
Protein 5,14g

# Almond Choc Cookies

## Ingredients
2 cups almond meal
1 1/2 tsp. almond extract
4 Tbsp. cocoa powder
5 Tbsp. coconut oil, melted
2 Tbsp. almond milk
4 Tbsp. agave nectar
2 tsp. vanilla extract
1/8 tsp. baking soda
1/8 tsp. salt

## Directions
1. Preheat oven to 340F degrees.
2. In a deep bowl mix salt, cocoa powder, almond meal and baking soda.
3. In a separate bowl, whisk together melted coconut oil, almond milk, almond and vanilla extract and maple syrup. Merge the almond meal mixture with almond milk mixture and mix well.
4. In a greased baking pan pour the batter evenly. Bake for 10-15 minutes. 5. Once ready let cool on a wire rack and serve.

Servings: 12

## Cooking Times
Total Time: 25 minutes

## Nutrition Facts (per serving)
Calories 79
Fat 5,94g
Carbs 7,02g
Fiber 0,61g
Protein 0,46g

# Carrot Flowers Muffins

**Ingredients**

2 eggs

2 cups shredded carrots

1/4 cup coconut flour

1/2 cup coconut oil

1 tsp. vanilla extract

1/4 cup Erythritol

2 tsp. ground cinnamon

1 tsp. baking powder

**Directions**

1. Preheat oven to 350F. Prepare12 muffin tins.
2. In your food processor, add in carrots, eggs, coconut oil, Erythritol, and vanilla. Blend together until combined.
3. In a separate bowl, mix together coconut flour, cinnamon and baking powder.
4. Pour the carrot mixture into the dry ingredients and mix until completely combined.
5. Pour carrot mixture into the muffin tin and bake for about 30-35 minutes.
6. Remove from the oven, and let cool for at least 30 minutes. Serve.

Servings: 12

**Cooking Times**

Total Time: 50 minutes

**Nutrition Facts (per serving)**

Calories 127

Fat 10,04g

Carbs 8,81g

Fiber 0,91g

Protein 1,53g

# Coconut Jelly Cake

**Ingredients**
1 cup coconut flour
1/2 cup butter, softened
2 Tbsp. raspberry jelly
1/2 cup coconut sugar
3 cups desiccated coconut
1 egg
2/3 cup coconut milk
1 cup boiling water
1 cup cold water
1/2 cup double thick cream

**Directions**
1. Preheat oven to 360F. Grease a patty pan.
2. In a bowl beat butter and coconut sugar until light. Add in egg and beat until well combined. Gently fold in half the coconut flour and half the milk. Repeat with remaining flour and milk.
3. Spoon mixture into patty pan. Bake for 15 to 20 minutes. Once ready, let cool cakes on a wire rack.
4. Stir jelly and boiling water together in a bowl until crystals are dissolved. Stir in cold water. Refrigerate for 1 hour.
5. Place coconut into a large bowl. Cut each cake in half. Stick halves back together using 1 teaspoon of cream. Using a slotted spoon lower cakes, 1 cake at a time, into jelly. Drain excess jelly.
6. Toss cakes in coconut until well coated. When ready, place onto a lined tray and refrigerate at least 1 hour or until set.

Servings: 18
**Cooking Time**: 30 minutes

**Nutrition Facts (per serving)**
Calories 146
Fat 14,31g
Carbs 4,21g
Fiber 2,16g
Protein 1,83g

# Cottage Pumpkin Pie Ice Cream

**Ingredients**
1/2 cup toasted pecans, chopped
3 egg yolks
2 Tbsp. butter, salted
2 cups coconut milk
1/2 cup pumpkin puree
1 tsp. pumpkin spice
1/2 cup cottage cheese
1/2 tsp. chia seeds
1/3 cup Erythritol
20 drops liquid Nutria

**Directions**
1. Place all ingredients into a container of your immersion blender. Blend all of the ingredients together into a smooth mixture.
2. Add mixture to your ice cream machine, as per instructions of your manufacturer.
3. Follow the churning instructions as per your ice cream maker manufacturer's instructions. Serve in a chilled bowls or glasses.

Servings: 6

**Cooking Times**
Total Time: 15 minutes

**Nutrition Facts (per serving)**
Calories 233
Fat 21,74g
Carbs 6,87g
Fiber 1,95g
Protein 5,49g

# Divine Chocolate Biscotti

**Ingredients**

1 egg

2 cups whole almonds

2 Tbsp. flax seeds

1 cup shredded coconut, unsweetened

1 cup coconut oil

1 cup cacao powder

1/4 cup Xylitol or Stevia sweetener

1 tsp. salt

1 tsp. baking soda

**Directions**

1. Preheat oven to 350F.
2. In a food process blend the whole almonds with the flax seeds. Add in the rest of ingredients and mix well.
3. Place the dough on a piece of aluminum foil to shape into 8 biscotti-shaped slices. Bake for 12 minutes.
4. Let cool and serve.

Servings: 8

**Cooking Times**

Total Time: 25 minutes

**Nutrition Facts (per serving)**

Calories 276

Fat 25,44g

Carbs 9,19g

Fiber 5,2g

Protein 8,24g

# Hemp and Chia Seeds Cream

**Ingredients**

1 ¼ cup coconut milk

2 Tbsp. hemp powder

2 sheets of unflavored gelatin

3 Tbsp. chia seeds

**Directions**

1.  In a saucepan over low heat add the coconut milk and dissolve the lucuma powder.
2.  Cut the gelatin into pieces and add it to the milk. Stir until dissolved completely.
3.  Add chia seeds and stir occasionally until mixture thickens, about 15 minutes.
4.  Pour the mixture into individual containers and allow cool before putting them in the refrigerator for at least 2 hours before serving.
5.  Enjoy!

Servings: 3

Cooking Time: 20 minutes

**Nutrition Facts (per serving)**

Calories 202

Fat 19,2g

Carbs 8,12g

Fiber 3,14g

Protein 2,59g

# Homemade Nuts Bars

**Ingredients**

1 cup almonds

1/2 cup hazelnut, chopped

1 cup peanuts

1 cup shredded coconut

1 cup almond butter

1 cup Liquid Erythritol

1 cup coconut oil, freshly melted and still warm

**Directions**

1. In a food processor place all nuts and chop for 1-2 minutes.
2. Add in grated coconut, almond butter, Erythritol and coconut oil. Process it for 1 minute about.
3. Cover a square bowl with parchment paper and place the mixture on top.
4. Flatten the mixture with a spatula. Place the bowl in the freezer for 4-5 hours.
5. Remove batter from the freezer, cut and serve.

Servings: 10

**Cooking Times**

Cooking Time: 10 minutes

Inactive Time: 5 hours

**Nutrition Facts (per serving)**

Calories 193

Fat 18,2g

Carbs 6,64g

Fiber 2,53g

Protein 3,83g

# Caramel Coffee Smoothie

**Ingredients**
1/2 cup heavy cream
1/2 cup almond milk, unsweetened
3 Tbsp. sugar-free chocolate syrup
3 Tbsp. sugar-free caramel syrup
3/4 cup cold coffee
2 Tbsp. cocoa, unsweetened
Ice cubes

**Directions**
1.  In a blender add all ingredients and blend until all incorporate well.
2.  Pour in glasses and serve.

Servings: 4

**Cooking Times**
Total Time: 5 minutes

**Nutrition Facts (per serving)**
Calories 170
Fat 14,95g
Carbs 9,02g
Fiber 1,92g
Protein 2,8g

# Chocolate Chia Cream

**Ingredients**
1/4 cup Chia seeds
1 cup heavy whipping cream
1 cup coconut milk
2 Tbsp. cocoa powder
pure vanilla extract
1/4 cup Erythritol sweetener

**Directions**
1. In a bowl mix the chia seeds and add the coconut milk until it combines well.
2. Add the Erythritol and whisk some more. Divide the mixture into two portions.
3. Add cocoa to one half and mixed it nicely.
4. Pour chia seed mixture into the bowls or glasses. Keep covered in the refrigerator for 12 hours.
1. Before serving beat the heavy whipping cream and pour over the chia seeds cream. Enjoy!

Servings: 4

**Cooking Times**
Total Time: 12 hours

**Nutrition Facts (per serving)**
Calories 341
Fat 35,41g
Carbs 7,35g
Fiber 1,56g
Protein 2,99g

# Chocolate Brownies

**Ingredients**
2 eggs
1 1/2 cups almond flour
1/4 cup coconut oil
1/2 cup cocoa powder, unsweetened
1 Tbsp. Metamucil Fiber Powder
1/3 cup Natvia (or some other natural sweetener)
1/4 cup maple syrup
1 tsp. baking powder
1/2 tsp. salt

**Directions**
1. Preheat oven to 350F.
2. In a bowl add in all wet ingredients and 2 Eggs. Beat the wet ingredients together using a hand mixer until a consistent mixture is formed.
3. In a separate bowl, combine all dry ingredients. Mix the dry ingredients well. Pour the wet ingredients slowly into the dry ingredients, mixing with a hand mixer as you pour.
4. Pour the batter into baking pan. Bake the brownies for 20 minutes.
5. When ready, let the brownies cool. Slice brownies into slices and serve.

Servings: 10

Cooking Times
Total Time: 35 minutes

**Nutrition Facts (per serving)**
Calories 157
Fat 13,4g
Carbs 8,07g
Fiber 2,58g
Protein 5,04g

# Chocolate Pecan Bites

**Ingredients**

2 oz. 100% dark chocolate

2.5 oz. pecan halves

cinnamon

nutmeg

**Directions**

1. Preheat oven to 350F.
2. Place the pecan halves on a parchment paper and bake in oven for 6-7 minutes. When ready, let cool and set aside.
3. Melt the dark chocolate.
4. Dip each pecan half in the melted dark chocolate and place back on the parchment paper.
5. Sprinkle a cinnamon and nutmeg on top of the chocolate covered pecans.
6. Before serving place in refrigerator for 2-3 hours.

Servings: 12

Cooking Time: 3 hours

**Nutrition Facts (per serving)**

Calories 52

Fat 4,96g

Carbs 2,32g

Fiber 0,71g

Protein 0,64g

# Hazelnuts Chocolate Cream

**Ingredients**

1 cup hazelnuts halves

4 Tbsp. unsweetened cocoa powder

1 tsp. pure vanilla extract

2 Tbsp. coconut oil

4 Tbsp. granulated Stevia (or sweetener of choice)

**Directions**

1. Place all the ingredients in your blender. Blend until smooth well.
2. Store in the fridge for 1 hour. Serve and enjoy!

Servings: 4

Cooking Times

Total Time: 5 minutes

**Nutrition Facts (per serving)**

Calories 302

Fat 29,65g

Carbs 9,5g

Fiber 5,12g

Protein 6,39g

# Instant Coffee Ice Cream

**Ingredients**
1 Tbsp. Instant Coffee
2 Tbsp. Cocoa Powder
1 cup coconut milk
1/4 cup heavy cream
1/4 tsp. flax seeds
2 Tbsp. Erythritol
15 drops liquid Nutria

**Directions**
1. Add all ingredients except the flax seeds into a container of your immersion blender.
2. Blend well until all ingredients are incorporated well. Slowly add in flax seeds until a slightly thicker mixture is formed. Add the mass to your ice cream machine and follow manufacturer's instructions.
3. Ready! Serve!

Servings: 2

Cooking Times
Total Time: 20 minutes

**Nutrition Facts (per serving)**
Calories 286
Fat 29,21g
Carbs 9,39g
Fiber 1,88g
Protein 3,18g

# Jam "Eye" Cookies

**Ingredients**
2 eggs
1 cup almond flour
2 Tbsp. coconut flour
2 Tbsp. sugar-free jam per taste
1/2 cup natural sweetener (Stevia, Truvia, Erythritol...etc.)
4 Tbsp. coconut oil
1/2 tsp. pure vanilla extract
1/2 tsp. almond extract
1 Tbsp. shredded coconut
1/2 tsp. baking powder
1/4 tsp. cinnamon
1/2 tsp. salt

**Directions**
1. Preheat your oven to 350F. In a big bowl, combine all your dry ingredients and whisk.
2. Add in your wet ingredients and combine well using hand mixer or a whisk.
3. With your hand for make the patties and place the cookies on a parchment paper lined baking sheet. Using your finger make an indent in the middle if each cookie.
4. Bake for about 16 minutes or until the cookies turn golden.
5. Once ready, let the cookies cool on a wire rack and fill each indent with sugar free jam.
6. Before serving sprinkle some shredded coconut on top of each cookie. Enjoy!

Servings: 16
**Cooking Times**: 36 minutes

**Nutrition Facts (per serving)**
Calories 95
Fat 8,61g
Carbs 2,79g
Fiber 1,02g
Protein 2, 71

# Lemon Coconut Pearls

**Ingredients**
3 packages of True Lemon (Crystallized Citrus for Water)
1/4 cup shredded coconut, unsweetened
1 cup cream cheese
1/4 cup granulated Stevia

**Directions**
1. In a bowl, combine cream cheese, lemon and Stevia. Blend well until incorporate.
2. Once the mixture is well combined, put it back in the fridge to harden up a bit.
3. Roll into 16 balls and dip each ball into shredded coconut. Refrigerate for several hours. Serve.

Servings: 4

Cooking Time: 15 minutes

**Nutrition Facts (per serving)**
Calories 216
Fat 21,53g
Carbs 3,12g
Fiber 0,45g
Protein 3,61g

# Lime & Vanilla Cheesecake

**Ingredients**

1/4 cup cream cheese, softened

2 Tbsp. heavy cream

1 tsp. lime juice

1 egg

1 tsp. pure vanilla extract

2-4 Tbsp. Erythritol or Stevia

**Directions**

1. In a microwave-safe bowl combine all ingredients. Place in a microwave and cook on HIGH for 90 seconds.
2. Every 30 seconds stir to combine the ingredients well.
3. Transfer mixture to a bowl and refrigerate for at least 2 hours.
4. Before serving top with whipped cream or coconut powder.

Servings: 2

Preparation Time: 5 minutes

Inactive Time: 2 hours

**Nutrition Facts (per serving)**

Calories 140

Fat 13g

Carbs 1,38g

Fiber 0,01g

Protein 4,34g

# Chocolate Mousse

**Ingredients**
1/4 cup of heavy cream
1 1/4 cup coconut cream
2 Tbsp. of cocoa powder
3 Tbsp. of Erythritol (or Stevia)
1 Tbsp. pure vanilla essence
shredded coconut, unsweetened

**Directions**
1. Scoop out the hardened coconut cream from the can, leaving the clear liquid behind, and place into a bowl. Add the heavy cream and combine with a hand mixer on low speed.
2. Add the remaining ingredients and mix on low speed for 2-3 minutes until the mix is thick.
3. Serve in individual ramekins sprinkled with unsweetened shredded coconut.

Servings: 4
Cooking Times: 15 minutes

**Nutrition Facts (per serving)**
Calories 305
Fat 31,91g
Carbs 6,97g
Fiber 2,55g
Protein 3,56g

# Strawberry Pudding

**Ingredients**
4 egg yolks
2 Tbsp. butter
1/4 cup coconut flour
2 Tbsp. heavy cream
1/4 cup strawberries
1/4 tsp. baking powder
2 Tbsp. coconut oil
2 tsp. lemon juice
Zest 1 Lemon
2 Tbsp. Erythritol
10 drops Liquid Stevia

**Directions**
1. Preheat oven to 350F.
2. In a bowl beat the egg yolks with electric mixer until they're pale in color. Add in Erythritol and 10 drops liquid Stevia. Beat again until fully combined.
3. Add in heavy cream, lemon juice, and the zest of 1 lemon. Add the coconut and butter. Beat well until no lumps are found.
4. Sift the dry ingredients over the wet ingredients, and then mix well on a slow speed.
5. Distribute the strawberries evenly in the batter by pushing them into the top of the batter.
6. Bake for 20-25 minutes. Once finished, let cool and serve.

Servings: 3

Cooking Times
Total Time: 35 minutes

**Nutrition Facts (per serving)**
Calories 258
Fat 23,46g
Carbs 9,3g
Fiber 0,61g
Protein 3,98g

# Kiwi Fiend Ice Cream

**Ingredients**
3 egg yolks
1 1/2 cup Kiwi, pureed
1 cup heavy cream
1/3 cup Erythritol
1/2 tsp. pure vanilla extract
1/8 tsp. chia seeds

**Directions**
1. In a sauce pan heat up the heavy cream. Add in 1/3 cup of erythritol to dissolve; simmer gently until erythritol is dissolved.
2. In a mixing bowl beat 3 egg yolks with an electric mixer. Add in a few tablespoons of your hot cream mixture at a time to the eggs while beating. Add in some pure vanilla extract and mix. Add in 1/8 tsp. of chia seeds.
3. Place your bowl into the freezer to chill for about 1-2 hours, stirring occasionally.
4. In a meanwhile puree the kiwi no more than 1-2 seconds. When the ice cream is chilled and getting a bit thicker, add in kiwi mixture to the chilled cream. Mix a bit.
5. Let the kiwi ice cream to chill at least 6-8 hours. Serve in chilled glasses.

Servings: 6

**Cooking Times**
Cooking Time: 15 minutes
Total Time: 8 hours and 15 minutes

**Nutrition Facts (per serving)**
Calories 192
Fat 17,2g
Carbs 8,13g
Fiber 1,46g
Protein 2,69g

# Minty Avocado Lime Sorbet

**Ingredients**
1 cup coconut milk
2 avocados
1/4 mint leaves, chopped
1/4 cup powdered Erythritol
2 limes, juiced
1/4 tsp. liquid Stevia

**Directions**
1.  Slice avocado half vertically through the flesh, making about 5 slices per half of an avocado. Use a spoon to carefully scoop out the pieces. Rest pieces on foil and squeeze juice of 1/2 lime over the tops.
2.  Store avocado in freezer for at least 3 hours.
3.  Using a spice grinder, powder Erythritol.
4.  In a pan, bring coconut milk to a boil.
5.  Zest the 2 limes you have while coconut milk is heating up. Add lime zest and continue to let the milk reduce in volume.
6.  Remove and place the coconut milk into a container and store in the freezer.
7.  Chop mint leaves. Remove avocados from freezer.
8.  Add avocado, mint leaves, and juice from lime into the food processor. Pulse until a chunky consistency is achieved.
9.  Pour coconut milk mixture over the avocados in the food processor. Add Liquid Stevia to this.
10. Pulse mixture together about 2-3 minutes.
11. Return to freezer to freeze, or serve immediately!

Servings: 6
**Cooking Times**: 3 hours and 15 minutes

**Nutrition Facts (per serving)**
Calories 184
Fat 17,26g
Carbs 9,65g
Fiber 4,59g
Protein 1,95g

# Morning Zephyr Cake

**Ingredients**

3 Tbsp. coconut oil

2 Tbsp. grounded flax seeds

8 Tbsp. almonds, grounded

1 cup Greek Yogurt

1 Tbsp. cocoa powder for dusting

1 cup heavy whipping cream

1 tsp. Baking Powder

1 tsp. Baking Soda

1 tsp. pure vanilla essence

1 pinch pink salt

1 cup Stevia or Erythritol sweetener

**Directions**

1. Pre-heat the oven at 350 F degrees.
2. In the blender first add the grounded almonds, grounded flax seeds and the baking powder and soda. Blend for a minute.
3. Add the salt, coconut oil and blend some more. Add the sweetener and blend for 2-3 minutes.
4. Add the Greek yogurt and blend for a minute or so, until a fine consistency is reached.
5. Take out the batter in a bowl and add the vanilla essence, and mix with a light hand.
6. Grease the baking dish and drop the batter in it.
7. Bake for 30 minutes. Let cool on a wire rack. Serve.

Servings: 8

**Cooking Times**

Total Time: 40 minutes

**Nutrition Facts (per serving)**

Calories 199

Fat 20,69g

Carbs 3,22g

Fiber 1,17g

Protein 2,56g

# Peanut Butter Balls

**Ingredients**

2 eggs

2 1/2 cup of peanut butter

1/2 cup shredded coconut (unsweetened)

1/2 cup of Xylitol

1 Tbsp. of pure vanilla extract

**Directions**

1. Preheat oven to 320 F.
2. Mix all ingredients together by your hands.
3. After the ingredients are thoroughly mixed, roll into heaped tablespoon sized balls and press into a baking tray lined with baking paper.
4. Bake in the oven for 12 minutes or until the tops of the cookies are browning. When ready, let cool on a wire rack. Ready! Serve.

Servings: 16

Cooking Time: 22 minutes

**Nutrition Facts (per serving)**

Calories 254

Fat 21,75g

Carbs 8,31g

Fiber 2,64g

Protein 10,98g

# Peppermint Chocolate Ice Cream

## Ingredients
1/2 tsp. Peppermint extract
1 cup heavy cream
1 cup cheese cream
1 tsp. pure vanilla extract
1 tsp. Liquid Stevia extract
100% Dark Chocolate for topping

## Directions
1. Place ice cream bowl in freezer per ice cream maker instructions. In a metal bowl, put all ingredients except chocolate and whisk well.
2. Put back in freezer for 5 minutes. Setup ice cream maker and add liquid.
3. Before serving, top the ice cream with chocolate shavings. Serve.

Servings: 3
Cooking Time: 35 minutes

## Nutrition Facts (per serving)
Calories 286
Fat 29,96g
Carbs 2,7g
Fiber 0g
Protein 2,6g

# Raspberry Chocolate Cream

## Ingredients
1/2 cup 100% dark chocolate, chopped
1/4 cup of heavy cream
1/2 cup cream cheese, softened
2 Tbsp. sugar free Raspberry Syrup
1/4 cup Erythritol

## Directions
1. In a double boiler melt chopped chocolate and the cream cheese. Add the Erythritol sweetener and continue to stir. Remove from heat, let cool and set aside.
2. When the cream has cooled add in heavy cream and Raspberry syrup and stir well.
3. Pour cream in a bowls or glasses and serve. Keep refrigerated.

Servings: 4
Cooking Time: 15 minutes

## Nutrition Facts (per serving)
Calories 157
Fat 13,51g
Carbs 7,47g
Fiber 1g
Protein 1,95g

# Raw Cacao Hazelnut Cookies

### Ingredients
2 cups almond flour
1 cup chopped hazelnut
1/2 cup cacao powder
1/2 cup ground flax
3 Tbsp. coconut oil (melted)
1/3 cup water
1/3 cup Erythritol
1/4 tsp. liquid Stevia

### Directions
1.  In a bowl, mix almond flour and flax and cacao powder. Stir in oil, water, agave and vanilla. When it is well mixed, stir in chopped hazelnuts.
2.  Form in to balls, press flat with palms and place on dehydrator screens.
3.  Dehydrate 1 hour at 145, then reduce to 116 and dehydrate for at least 5 hours or until desired dryness is achieved.
4.  Serve.

Servings: 24
Cooking Time: 6 hours

### Nutrition Facts (per serving)
Calories 181
Fat 15,69g
Carbs 8,75g
Fiber 3,45g
Protein 4,46g

# Sinless Pumpkin Cheesecake Muffins

**Ingredients**

1/2 cup pureed pumpkin

1 tsp. pumpkin pie spice

1/2 cup pecans, finely ground

1/2 cup cream cheese

1 Tbsp. coconut oil

1/2 tsp. pure vanilla extract

1/4 tsp. pure Yacon Syrup or Erythritol

**Directions**

1. Prepare a muffin tin with liners.
2. Place a small amount of ground pecans into every muffin tin and make a thin crust.
3. In a bowl, blend sweetener, spices, vanilla, coconut and the pumpkin puree. Add in the cream cheese and beat until the mixture is well combined.
4. Scoop about two tablespoons of filling mixture on top of each crust, and smooth around the edges.
5. Pop in the freezer for about 45 minutes.
6. Remove from the muffin tin and let sit for 10 minutes. Serve.

Servings: 6

Cooking Times
Total Time: 15 minutes

**Nutrition Facts (per serving)**

Calories 157

Fat 15,52g

Carbs 3,94g

Fiber 1,51g

Protein 2,22g

# Hazelnut Biscuits with Arrowroot Tea

**Ingredients**

1 egg

1/2 cup hazelnuts

3 Tbsp. of coconut oil

2 cups almond flour

2 Tbsp. of arrowroot tea

2 tsp. ginger

1 Tbsp. cocoa powder

1/2 cup grapefruit juice

1 orange peel from a half orange

1/2 tsp. baking soda

1 pinch of salt

**Directions**

1. Preheat oven to 360 °F. Make arrowroot tea and let it cool.
2. In a food processor blend the hazelnuts. Add the remaining ingredients and continue blending until mixed well. With your hands form cookies with the batter.
3. Put the cookies on baking parchment paper, and bake for 30-35 minutes. When ready, remove tray from the oven and let cool.
4. Serve warm or cold.

Servings: 12

**Cooking Times**

Total Time: 50 minutes

**Nutrition Facts (per serving)**

Calories 224

Fat 20,17g

Carbs 8,06g

Fiber 3,25g

Protein 6,36g

# Tartar Cookies

## Ingredients
3 eggs
1/8 tsp. cream of tartar
1/3 cup cream cheese
1/8 tsp. salt
Some oil for greasing

## Directions
1.  Preheat oven to 300°F. Line the cookie sheet with parchment paper and grease with some oil.
2.  Separate eggs from the egg yolks. Set both in different mixing bowls.
3.  With an electric hand mixer, start beating the egg whites until super bubbly. Add in cream of tartar and beat until stiff peaks form.
4.  In the egg yolk bowl, add in cream cheese and some salt. Beat until the egg yolks are pale yellow.
5.  Merge the egg whites into the cream cheese mixture. Stir well.
6.  Make cookies and place on the cookie sheet.
7.  Bake for about 30-40 minutes. When ready, let them cool on a wire rack and serve.

Servings: 8

## Cooking Times
Total Time: 35 minutes

## Nutrition Facts (per serving)
Calories 59,
Fat 5,09g
Carbs 0,56g
Fiber 0g
Protein 2,93g

# Wild Strawberries Ice Cream

**Ingredients**
1/2 cup wild strawberries
1/3 cup cream cheese
1 cup heavy cream
1 Tbsp. lemon juice
1 tsp. pure vanilla extract
1/3 cup of your favorite sweetener
Ice cubes

**Directions**
1. Place all ingredients in a blender. Blend until all incorporate well.
2. Refrigerate for 2-3 hour before serving.

Servings: 4
Cooking Time: 5 minutes

**Nutrition Facts (per serving)**
Calories 176
Fat 17,69g
Carbs 3,37g
Fiber 0,39g
Protein 1,9g

# Mini Lemon Cheesecakes

## Ingredients

1 tablespoon lemon zest, grated
1 teaspoon lemon juice
½ teaspoon stevia powder or (Truvia)
1/4 cup coconut oil, softened
4 tablespoons unsalted butter, softened
4 ounces cream cheese (heavy cream)

## Directions

1. Blend all ingredients together with a hand mixer or blender until smooth and creamy.
2. Prepare a cupcake or muffin tin with 6 paper liners.
3. Pour mixture into prepared tin and place in freezer for 2-3 hours or until firm.
4. Sprinkle cups with additional lemon zest. Or try using chopped nuts or shredded, unsweetened coconut.

Serves: 6
Cooking Time: 5 minutes

## Nutrition Facts (per serving)

Calories: 196
Fat: 21.2 grams

# Chocolate Layered Coconut Cups

### Ingredients

Bottom Layer:

1/2 cup unsweetened, shredded coconut

3 tablespoons powdered sweetener such as Splenda or Truvia

1/2 cup coconut butter

1/2 cup coconut oil

Top Layer:

1 1/2 ounces cocoa butter

1 ounce unsweetened chocolate

1/4 cup cocoa powder

1/2 teaspoon vanilla extract

1/4 cup powdered sweetener such as Splenda or Truvia

### Directions

1. Prepare a mini-muffin pan with 20 mini paper liners.
2. For the bottom layer:
3. Combine coconut butter and coconut oil in a small saucepan over low heat. Stir until smooth and melted then add the shredded coconut and powdered sweetener until combined.
4. Divide the mixture among prepared mini muffin cups and freeze until firm, about 30 minutes.
5. For the top layer:
6. Combine cocoa butter and unsweetened chocolate together in double boiler or a bowl set over a pan of simmering water. Stir until melted.
7. Stir in the powdered sweetener, then the cocoa powder and mix until smooth. Remove from heat and stir in the vanilla extract.
8. Spoon chocolate topping over chilled coconut candies and let set, about 15 minutes. Enjoy!

Serves: 10

Serving Size: 2 pieces

### Nutrition Facts (per serving)

Calories: 240

Fat: 25 grams

# Pumpkin Pie Chocolate Cups

**Ingredients**

For the crust:
3.5 ounces extra dark chocolate - 85% cocoa solids or more
2 tablespoons coconut oil

For the pie:
½ cup coconut butter
¼ cup coconut oil
2 teaspoons pumpkin pie spice mix
½ cup unsweetened pumpkin puree
2 tablespoons healthy low-carb sweetener
Optional: 15-20 drops liquid stevia for added sweetness

**Directions**
1. Place the chocolate and coconut oil in a double boiler or a glass bowl on top of a small saucepan filled with simmering water. Once completely melted, remove from the heat and set aside.
2. Prepare a mini muffin tin with 18 paper liners. Fill each of the 18 mini muffin cups with 2 teaspoons of the chocolate mixture. Place the chocolate in the fridge to set up for at least 10 minutes.
3. Place the coconut butter, coconut oil, sweetener and pumpkin spice mix into a bowl and melt just like you did the chocolate.
4. Add the pumpkin puree and mix until smooth and well combined.
5. Remove the muffin cups from the fridge and add a heaping teaspoon of the pumpkin & coconut mixture into every cup. Place back in the fridge and let it set for at least 30 minutes.
6. When done, keep refrigerated. Coconut oil and butter get very soft at room temperature. Store in the fridge for up to a week or freeze for up to 3 months. Enjoy!

Serves: 18
Serving Size: 1 mini pie

**Nutrition Facts (per serving)**
Calories: 110
Fat: 10.9 grams

# Fudgy Slow Cooker Cake

**Ingredients**
1 1/2 cups almond flour
1/4 cup whey protein powder (chocolate, vanilla, and unflavored all work fine)
3/4 cup sugar substitute such as Swerve or Truvia
2/3 cup cocoa powder
2 teaspoons baking powder
1/4 teaspoon sea salt
1/2 cup butter, melted
4 large eggs
3/4 cup almond or coconut milk, unsweetened
1 teaspoon vanilla extract
1/2 cup chopped dark chocolate, 85% cocoa or higher

Whipped cream topping (optional):
1/2 cup heavy whipping cream
2 tablespoons sugar substitute

**Directions**
1.    Grease the insert of a 6 quart slow cooker with butter or coconut oil.
2.    In a medium bowl, whisk together almond flour, sugar substitute, cocoa powder, whey protein powder, baking powder and salt.
3.    Stir in butter, eggs, almond milk and vanilla extract until well combined, then fold in the chopped dark chocolate.
4.    Pour into the greased slow cooker and cook on low for 2.5 to 3 hours. It will be gooey and like a pudding cake at 2.5 hours and little more cake like at 3 hours.
5.    Turn slow cooker off and let cool for 20 to 30 minutes. Cut into pieces and serve warm.
6.    Best when served with freshly whipped cream. To make this, mix the whipping cream and sugar substitute together with your stand mixer, or a hand mixer. Continue mixing until soft peaks form.

Serves: 10
Serving Size: 1/10th of cake

**Nutrition Facts (per serving)**
Calories: 275
Fat: 23

**314**

# Easy Sticky Chocolate Fudge

## Ingredients
1 cup coconut oil, softened
1/4 cup coconut milk (full fat, from a can)
1/4 cup cocoa powder
1 teaspoon vanilla extract
1/2 teaspoon sea salt
1-3 drops liquid stevia

## Directions
1.  With a hand mixer or stand mixer, whip the softened coconut oil and coconut milk together until smooth and glossy. About 6 minutes on high.
2.  Add the cocoa powder, vanilla extract, sea salt, and one drop of liquid stevia to the bowl and mix on low until combined. Increase speed once everything is combined and mix for one minute. Taste fudge and adjust sweetness by adding additional liquid stevia, if desired.
3.  Prepare a 9"x4" loaf pan by lining it with parchment paper.
4.  Pour fudge into loaf pan and place in freezer for about 15, until just set.
5.  Remove fudge and cut into 1" x 1" pieces. Store in an airtight container in the fridge or freezer.

Serves: 12

## Nutrition Facts (per serving)
Calories: 172
Fat: 19.6 grams

# Raspberry & Coconut Balls

### Ingredients

1/2 cup coconut butter

1/2 cup coconut oil

1/2 cup freeze dried raspberries

1/2 cup unsweetened shredded coconut

1/4 powdered sugar substitute such as Swerve or Truvia

### Directions

1. Line an 8"x8" pan with parchment paper.
2. In a food processor, coffee grinder, or blender, pulse the dried raspberries into a fine powder.
3. In a saucepan over medium heat, combine the coconut butter, coconut oil, coconut, and sweetener. Stir until melted and well combined.
4. Remove pan from heat and stir in raspberry powder.
5. Pour mixture into pan and refrigerate or freeze for several hours, or overnight.
6. Cut into 12 pieces and serve!

Serves: 12

Serving Size: 1 piece

### Nutrition Facts (per serving)

Calories: 234

Fat: 23.6 grams

# Strawberry Cheesecake Ice Cream Cups

**Ingredients**

1/2 strawberries, fresh or frozen, mashed well

3/4 cup cream cheese, softened

1/4 cup coconut oil, softened

10-15 drops liquid stevia

1 teaspoon vanilla extract

**Directions**

1. Combine all ingredients in a medium sized bowl and mix with a hand mixer until smooth and creamy. Can also be done in a food processor or high speed blender.)
2. Spoon the mixture into mini muffin silicon molds or small candy molds. Place in the freezer for about 2 hours or until set.
3. When done, unmold the fat bombs and place into a container. Keep in the freezer and enjoy any time!

Serves: 12

Serving Size: 1 bite

**Nutrition Facts (per serving)**

Calories: 67

Fat: 7.4 grams

# Peppermint Patties

### Ingredients
¾ cup melted coconut butter
¼ cup finely shredded, unsweetened coconut
2 tablespoons cacao powder
3 tablespoons coconut oil, melted
½ teaspoon pure peppermint extract

### Directions
1. Mix together melted coconut butter, shredded coconut, 1 tablespoon of coconut oil and peppermint extract
2. Pour coconut butter mixture into mini muffin tins that have been lined with paper liners. Fill half way.
3. Place in refrigerator and allow to harden for about 15 minutes.
4. Mix together 2 tablespoons coconut oil and cacao powder.
5. Remove muffin tin from refrigerator and top each one with chocolate mixture.
6. Return to refrigerator until the chocolate has set.
7. When ready to eat, simply set the peppermint patty cups on the counter for about 5 minutes and unmold from muffin tin.

Serves: 12

### Nutrition Facts (per serving)
Calories: 80
Fat: 7g

318

# Buttery Pecan Delights

**Ingredients**

8 pecan halves
1 tablespoon unsalted butter, softened
2 ounces neufchâtel cheese
1 teaspoon orange zest, finely grated
pinch of sea salt

**Directions**

1. Toast the pecans at 350 degrees Fahrenheit for 5-10 minutes, check often to prevent burning.
2. Mix the butter, neufchâtel cheese, and orange zest until smooth and creamy.
3. Spread the butter mixture between the cooled pecan halves and sandwich together.
4. Sprinkle with sea salt and enjoy!

Serves: 2
Serving Size: 2 pecan sandwiches

**Nutrition Facts (per serving)**
Calories: 163
Fat: 16 grams

# Fudge Oh So Chocolate

**Ingredients**

1 cup coconut oil, softened
1/4 cup coconut milk (full fat, from a can)
1/2 teaspoon sea salt
1-3 drops liquid stevia
1/4 cup cocoa powder
1 teaspoon vanilla extract

**Directions**

1. With a hand mixer or stand mixer, whip the softened coconut oil and coconut milk together until smooth and glossy. About 6 minutes on high.
2. Add the cocoa powder, vanilla extract, sea salt, and one drop of liquid stevia to the bowl and mix on low until combined. Increase speed once everything is combined and mix for one minute. Taste fudge and adjust sweetness by adding additional liquid stevia, if desired.
3. Prepare a 9"x4" loaf pan by lining it with parchment paper.
4. Pour fudge into loaf pan and place in freezer for about 15, until just set.
5. Remove fudge and cut into 1" x 1" pieces. Store in an airtight container in the fridge or freezer.

Serves: 12

**Nutrition Facts (per serving)**

Calories: 172
Fat: 19.6 grams

# Cinna-Bun Balls

## Ingredients

1 cup coconut butter

1 teaspoon vanilla extract

1 cup full fat coconut milk (from a can)

1 cup unsweetened coconut shreds

1/2 teaspoon cinnamon

1/2 teaspoon nutmeg

1 teaspoon sugar substitute such as Splenda

## Directions

1. Combine all ingredients except the shredded coconut together in double boiler or a bowl set over a pan of simmering water. Stir until everything is melted and combined.
2. Remove bowl from heat and place in the fridge until the mixture has firmed up and can be rolled into balls.
3. Form the mixture into 1" balls, a small cookie scoop is helpful for doing this.
4. Roll each ball in the shredded coconut until well coated.
5. Serve and enjoy! Store in the fridge.

Serves: 10

## Nutrition Facts (per serving)

Calories: 273

Fat: 30.9g

# Vanilla Mousse Cups

**Ingredients**
8 ounces (1 block) cream cheese, softened
1/2 cup sugar substitute such as Swerve or Truvia (Stevia)
1 1/2 teaspoons vanilla extract
dash of sea salt
1/2 cup heavy whipping cream

**Directions**
1. Add the first four ingredients to a food processor or blender.
2. Blend until combined.
3. With blender running, slowly add the heavy cream.
4. Continue to blend until thickened, about 1-2 minutes. Consistency should be mousse like.
5. Prepare a cupcake or muffin tin with 6 paper liners and portion the mixture into the cups.
6. Chill in the fridge until set and enjoy!

Serves: 6

**Nutrition Facts (per serving)**
Calories: 199
Fat: 20.2 grams

# Rich & Creamy Ice Cream

**Ingredients**
4 whole pastured eggs
4 yolks from pastured eggs
⅓ cup melted cocoa butter
⅓ cup melted coconut oil
15-20 drops liquid stevia
⅓ cup cocoa powder
¼ cup MCT oil
2 teaspoons pure vanilla extract
8-10 ice cubes

**Directions**
1. Add all ingredients but the ice cubes into the jug of your high speed blender. Blend on high for 2 minutes, until creamy.
2. While the blender is running, remove the top portion of the lid and drop in 1 ice cube at a time, allowing the blender to run about 10 seconds between each ice cube.
3. Once all of the ice has been added, pour the cold mixture into a 9×5" loaf pan and place in the freezer. Set the timer for 30 minutes before taking out to stir. Repeat this process for 2-3 hours, until desired consistency is met.
4. Serve immediately. Top with chopped nuts or shaved dark chocolate, if desired.
5. Store covered in the freezer for up to a week.

Serves: 5

Serving Size: 1 cup

**Nutrition Facts (per serving)**
Calories: 431
Fat: 44.3

# English Toffee Treats

### Ingredients
1 cup coconut oil
2 tablespoons butter
1/2 block cream cheese, softened
3/4 tablespoons cocoa powder
1/2 cup creamy, natural peanut butter
3 tablespoons Davinci Gourmet Sugar Free English Toffee Syrup

### Directions
1. Combine all ingredients in a saucepan over medium heat.
2. Stir until everything is smooth, melted, and combined.
3. Pour mixture into small candy molds or mini muffin tins lined with paper liners.
4. Freeze or refrigerate until set and enjoy!
5. Store in an airtight container in the fridge.

Serves: 24

Serving Size: 1 piece

### Nutrition Facts (per serving)
Calories: 142
Fat: 15 grams

# Fudgy Peanut Butter Squares

**Ingredients**

1 cup all natural creamy peanut butter

1 cup coconut oil

1/4 cup unsweetened vanilla almond milk

a pinch of coarse sea salt

1 teaspoon vanilla extract

2 teaspoons liquid stevia (optional)

**Directions**

1. In a microwave safe bowl, soften the peanut butter and coconut oil together. (About 1 minute on med-low heat.)
2. Combine the softened peanut butter and coconut oil with the remaining ingredients into a blender or food processor.
3. Blend until thoroughly combined.
4. Pour into a 9X4" loaf pan that has been lined with parchment paper.
5. Refrigerate until set. About 2 hours.
6. Enjoy!

Serves: 12

**Nutrition Facts (per serving)**

Calories: 287

Fat: 29.7

# Almond Butter Balls

### Ingredients
2 1/2 cup almond butter
1/2 cup shredded coconut (unsweetened)
2 eggs
1/2 cup Stevia sweetener
1 Tbsp. pure vanilla extract

### Directions
1. Preheat oven to 320 F. Line square baking tray with baking paper.
2. Place all ingredients in a bowl. Knead the mixture by your hands.
3. After the ingredients are mixed, roll into heaped teaspoon sized balls and place into a baking tray.
4. Bake in the oven for 12 minutes or until the tops of the cookies are browning. Let cool on a wire rack. Serve.

Servings: 24
Cooking Time: 22 minutes

### Nutrition Facts (per serving)
Carbs: 5,6g
Protein: 7,3g
Fat: 14,5g
Calories: 171

# Cheesy Hazelnut Morsels

**Ingredients**
1/2 cup ground hazelnuts
1/4 cup hazelnut butter
1 cup cream cheese
1/4 cup cocoa powder
2 Tbsp. Sugar free Hazelnut syrup
Natural sweetener of your cheese, to taste

**Directions**
1. In a large bowl, place the softened cream cheese (on room temperature) and hazelnut butter. Add in all other ingredients (except the ground hazelnuts).
2. With a wooden spoon to blend the cream cheese, cocoa powder, butter, syrup and sweetener.
3. In a bowl place the ground hazelnuts. Roll the cream cheese mixture into 16 balls. Dip each ball into the ground hazelnuts.
4. Refrigerate for at least 2-3 hours.

Servings: 16
Cooking Time: 15 minutes

**Nutrition Facts (per serving)**
Carbs: 3,4g
Fiber: 1,4g
Protein: 3,2g
Fat: 11,6g
Calories: 122

# Choco Mint Hazelnut Sticks

### Ingredients
4 Tbsp. cocoa powder
1 cup shredded coconut
1 cup hazelnuts
1 tsp. peppermint extract
6 Tbsp. coconut oil, melted
4 Tbsp. almond butter
3/4 cup Stevia sweetener (or some other natural sweetener of your choice)
1 tsp. vanilla extract
pinch of salt

### Directions
1. In a large bowl stir together the coconut oil, cacao powder, almond butter, sweetener, vanilla, peppermint extract and salt. Chop the hazelnuts in a food processor.
2. Heat the mixture slowly on low heat over simmering water (double boiler) for 5 to 10 minutes until all ingredients are combined well.
3. Add hazelnuts and shredded coconut to the melted chocolate mixture and stir together.
4. Pour in a dish lined with parchment and freeze until chocolate is set then cut into sticks.

Servings: 12

### Cooking Times
Total Time: 20 minutes

### Nutrition Facts (per serving)
Carbs: 5,6g
Fiber: 2,4g
Protein: 3g
Fat: 17g
Calories: 174

# Chocolate Bomb Cookies

## Ingredients

1 Tbsp. cacao powder
2 Tbsp. chocolate protein powder
4 Tbsp. coconut milk
2 Tbsp. coconut flour
2 Tbsp. coconut, shredded
1 Tbsp. cacao nibs
Topping
1 tsp. coconut oil, softened
2/3 cup coconut butter, softened

## Directions

1. In a bowl combine all ingredients (except ingredients for coating). Whisk 2-3 minutes until well combined.
2. Spoon out mixture into small molds.
3. Place molds in refrigerator for 30 minutes.
4. In a meanwhile prepare coating. In a bowl, mix coconut oil with coconut butter. Remove molds from refrigerator and cover with coating
5. Place back to refrigerator until coating has hardened, about 1 hour.

Servings: 10

Cooking Times
Total Time: 10 minutes

## Nutrition Facts (per serving)

Carbs: 2,55g
Fiber: 1g
Protein: 1g
Fat: 14,47g
Calories: 138

# Chocolate Peanut Butter Balls

**Ingredients**

1/2 stick butter, softened

1/2 cup natural peanut butter

2 Tbsp. coconut flour

2 Tbsp. vanilla whey protein powder

1/2 cup broken up sugar free chocolate bars, melted

1 tsp. organic vanilla extract

1 1/2 cup powdered Xylitol (or some other natural sweetener)

**Directions**

1. In a bowl, mix peanut butter and butter. Beat the butter with an electric hand mixer, beat together butter until smooth.
2. Add in vanilla extract and protein powder to peanut butter mixture, and then mix well.
3. Add in powdered Xylitol sweetener and mix well.
4. On a working surface, roll the dough into 24 two-bite sized balls. Place balls on a pan lined with a parchment paper.
5. Sprinkle each ball with chocolate. Refrigerate for at least 2 hours.

Servings: 12

**Cooking Times**

Total Time: 10 minutes

**Nutrition Facts (per serving)**

Carbs: 5,16g

Fiber: 1,02g

Protein: 3g

Fat: 12g

Calories: 126

# Choco-Orange Walnut Muffin Bombs

### Ingredients
1 1/2 cup walnuts, chopped
4.40 oz. dark chocolate, 100% cocoa
1 tsp. natural orange extract
1 tsp. fresh orange peel
4 Tbsp.p extra virgin coconut oil
15-20 drops of liquid Stevia
1 tsp. cinnamon

### Directions
1.  In a heated container of water (water bath) melt the chocolate stirring slightly. Add liquid Stevia, coconut oil and cinnamon. Mix well.
2.  Add fresh orange peel and natural orange extract. Add chopped walnuts and mix in well.
3.  When ready, with teaspoon place the mixture into small paper muffin.
4.  Place in the fridge until solid, at least 4-6 hours.

Servings: 18

### Cooking Times
Total Time: 20 minutes

### Nutrition Facts (per serving)
Carbs: 5g
Fiber: 1,5g
Protein: 13g
Fat: 13g
Calories: 131

# Cinnamon Storms

### Ingredients
1 cup coconut milk
1 cup almond butter
1 tsp. pure vanilla extract
3/4 tsp. cinnamon
1/2 tsp. nutmeg
1 tsp. natural sweetener to your taste)
1 cup coconut shreds

### Directions
1. In a double boiler over medium heat place all the ingredients (except shredded coconut). Stir all the time to melt and combine well.
2. When ready, remove from the heat. Let cool for 5-6 minutes. Place the bowl in the fridge about 45 minutes until hard.
3. In a bowl put the coconut shreds. Roll the coconut-cinnamon mixture into one inch balls and roll them through the coconut shreds.
4. Place the balls on a serving plate and refrigerate for 2-3 hours.

Servings: 12

### Cooking Times
Preparation Time: 1 hour and 30 minutes

### Nutrition Facts (per serving)
Carbs: 1,6g
Fiber: 0,5g
Protein: 1g
Fat: 20g
Calories: 184

# Creamy Orange Bites

## Ingredients

1/2 cup heavy whipping cream
1/2 cup cream cheese
1/2 cup coconut oil, melted
1 tsp. pure orange extract
10 drops Liquid Stevia (or the natural sweetener of your choice)

## Directions

1. In an immersion blender place all ingredients. Blend until corporate well.
2. Add in orange extract and liquid Stevia and mix together with a spoon.
3. Spread the batter mixture into a silicone tray, or in paper muffins trays.
4. Refrigerate for 2 hours. Before serving remove from silicone tray and serve. Keep refrigerated.

Servings: 14
Cooking Time: 10 minutes

## Nutrition Facts (per serving)

Carbs: 0,5g
Protein: 1g
Fat: 14g
Calories: 127

# Coco-Nut Bites

## Ingredients
1 1/2 cup flaked coconut, unsweetened
1 cup coconut oil
1 cup extra virgin coconut oil
1 tsp. cinnamon powder
1/8 tsp. salt
2 Tbsp. of powdered Erythritol

## Directions
1. Preheat the oven 350 F.
2. Arrange evenly the flaked coconut on a rectangular baking tray. Place in the oven and toast for 8 minutes strictly. Let cool 2-3 minutes.
3. Transfer baked coconut into a blender and pulse until get a smooth and runny consistency.
4. Add the softened coconut oil, vanilla, Erythritol, salt and cinnamon. Blend well.
5. Pour the mixture with the tablespoon into ice cube tray to get 12 servings. Refrigerate for at least 2-3 hours.
6. Ready. Serve and enjoy! Keep refrigerated.

Servings: 12

Cooking Times
Total Time: 15 minutes

## Nutrition Facts (per serving)
Carbs: 1,5g
Fiber: 1g
Protein: 0,4g
Fat: 13g
Calories: 114

# Easy Choco Blueberry Squares

## Ingredients
5 Tbsp. butter
3 Tbsp. coconut oil
2 Tbsp. sugar-free Blueberry syrup
2 Tbsp. cocoa powder

## Directions
1.  In a sauce pan add all ingredients and cook over low heat until chocolate sauce texture.
2.  Pour into mold and freeze for at least 3 hours.
3.  Before serving unmold and enjoy.

Servings: 6
Cooking Time: 15 minutes

## Nutrition Facts (per serving)
Carbs: 1g
Fiber: 0,6g
Protein: 0,5g
Fat: 17g
Calories: 148

# Easy Jello Balls

**Ingredients**

1 cup cream cheese

1/4 cup coconut butter

1 package of sugar free jello

**Directions**

1. In a small bowl put the jello powder.
2. In a separate bowl, mix together cream cheese and coconut butter.
3. Take a teaspoon of batter, roll into a ball in your hands and then roll in the jello powder. Make 16 balls.
4. Cover with plastic wrap and place in the fridge.

Servings: 8

Cooking Time 10 minutes

**Nutrition Facts (per serving)**

Carbs: 1,20g

Protein: 2g

Fat: 16g

Calories: 150g

# Gingery Coconut Bombs

**Ingredients**

1 tsp. dried (powdered) ginger

0.8 oz. shredded coconut (unsweetened)

1/3 cup coconut oil, softened

1/3 cup coconut butter, softened

1 tsp. granulated sweetener of choice, to taste

**Directions**

1.  In a deep bowl, mix shredded coconut, coconut oil, coconut butter, sweetener and dried powdered ginger.
2.  Pour the ginger mixture into ice block trays and refrigerate for 1 hour to solidify.

Servings: 10

Cooking Time: 5 minutes

**Nutrition Facts (per serving)**

Carbs: 2,5g

Protein:

Fat: 14,5g

Calories: 134

# Homemade Almond Butter

### Ingredients
3 cups almonds (no salt added)
1 tsp. Himalayan salt
1 tsp. cinnamon
1 vanilla pod or bean, halved and seeds removed
2 Tbsp. Stevia powder or Erythritol sweetener

### Directions
1. Preheat oven to 360F degrees. Place almonds in a baking pan and bake for 10-12 minutes. Stir occasionally to not burn.
2. Transfer the almonds in a food processor and add remaining ingredients.
3. Process for 15 minutes above. This process takes a time so, you have to be patient. Pour the almond butter to a glass container and store in the refrigerator.

Servings: 14

### Cooking Times
Total Time: 40 minutes

### Nutrition Facts (per serving)
Carbs: 5,5g
Fiber: 2,8g
Protein: 5g
Fat: 13,5g
Calories: 153g

# Almond Cookies

**Ingredients**

1 cup almonds, chopped

1 cup butter, softened

2 1/4 cups almond flour

1 1/4 cup cocoa powder

3 1/2 Tbsp. coconut flour

2 eggs

3/4 cup Stevia powder

2 tsp. vanilla extract

1/2 tsp. baking soda

1/4 tsp. sea salt

**Directions**

1. Preheat oven to 340F degrees.
2. In a bowl, whisk butter and sweetener. Add the eggs, coconut oil and vanilla extract.
3. In a separate bowl, mix together the baking soda, almond flour, coconut flour, cocoa powder and salt.
4. Combine the eggs mixture to the flour mixture. Pour dough in a greased baking pan. Sprinkle dough with chopped almond over top.
5. Bake for 15-18 minutes. Let cool and cut into chunks. Serve.

Servings: 16

**Cooking Times**

Total Time: 25 minutes

**Nutrition Facts (per serving)**

Carbs: 3,35g

Fiber: 1g

Protein: 2,9g

Fat: 17g

Calories: 171

# Chocolate & Hazelnut Squares

**Ingredients**
1/2 cup hazelnuts, chopped
1 cup whipped cream
1/4 cup cocoa butter
2 Tbsp. cocoa powder, unsweetened
2 Tbsp. Stevia sweetener
Crushed walnuts (optional extra)

**Directions**
1. In a bowl, melt cocoa butter at room temperature.
2. When ready, add in cocoa powder, Stevia powder and mix well until all ingredients are well blended. Add in chopped hazelnuts and stir well.
3. Finally, add whipping cream and mix well.
4. Pour the hazelnut mixture in squared molds and let cool. (ice trays work just fine)
5. Refrigerate for 1 - 2 hours. Dress with crushed walnuts if so desired Serve.

Servings: 6

**Cooking Times**
Total Time: 15 minutes

**Nutrition Facts (per serving)**
Carbs: 3,8g
Fiber: 1,3g
Protein: 2g
Fat: 16,5g
Calories: 160

# Lime Balls

**Ingredients**

fresh lime zest from 2 organic limes
1 cup extra virgin coconut oil, softened
3/4 cup coconut butter, softened
20 drops Erythritol extract (or some other natural sweetener of your choice)
pinch of salt

**Directions**

1. Soft the coconut butter and coconut oil on room temperature.
2. Zest the organic limes.
3. In a bowl mix all the ingredients in a bowl and stir well. Make sure that lime zest and Erythritol extract are distributed evenly.
4. Prepare 16 mini muffin cups.
5. Refrigerate for 2 hours. Ready. Keep refrigerated.

Servings: 16

**Cooking Times**

Total Time: 10 minutes

**Nutrition Facts (per serving)**

Carbs: 0,9g
Fiber: 0,3g
Protein: 0,2g
Fat: 12,5g
Calories: 109

# Lemon Coconut Balls

### Ingredients
1/4 cup shredded coconut, unsweetened,
1 cup cream cheese
1 Tbsp. pure lemon extract
Natural sweetener of your choice, to taste
1/4 cup butter

### Directions
1.  In a bowl, combine cream cheese, natural sweetener and lemon extract. Blend all ingredients together well with mixing spoon. Place bowl in refrigerator for 15-20 minutes.
2.  In a bowl place unsweetened shredded coconut. Roll lemon batter into 16 equal balls.
3.  Dip each ball into coconut and place on a serving pan. Refrigerate for 3-4 hours at least. Serve.

Servings: 12
Cooking Time: 15 minutes

### Nutrition Facts (per serving)
Carbs: 1g
Protein: 1,3g
Fat: 12g
Calories: 106

# Heavenly Lemon Quads with Coconut Cream

**Ingredients**
Base
3/4 cup coconut flakes
2 Tbsp. coconut oil
1 Tbsp. ground almonds

Cream
5 eggs
1/2 lemon juice
1 Tbsp. coconut flour
1/2 cup Stevia sweetener

**Directions**
For the Base
1. Preheat oven to 360F.
2. In a bowl put all base ingredients and with clean hands mix everything well until soft.
3. With coconut oil grease a rectangle oven dish. Pour dough in a baking pan. Bake for 15 minutes until golden brown. Set aside to cool.

For the Cream
1. In a bowl or blender, whisk together: eggs, lemon juice, coconut flour and sweetener. Pour over the baked caked evenly.
2. Put pan in the oven and bake 20 minutes more.
3. When ready refrigerate for at least 6 hours. Cut in cubes and serve.

Servings: 8
**Cooking Times**: 1 hour and 5 minutes

**Nutrition Facts (per serving)**
Carbs: 4g
Fiber: 2,25g
Protein: 5g
Fat: 15g
Calories: 129

343

# Macadamia Cacao Cookies

**Ingredients**
1 cup macadamia nuts, chopped
1/2 cup cacao powder
2 cups almond flour
1/2 cup ground flax
3 Tbsp. coconut oil (melted)
1/3 cup Stevia or natural sweetener of your choice
1/3 cup water
1/2 tsp. pure vanilla extract

**Directions**
1. In a bowl, mix almond flour and flax and cacao powder. Stir in oil, water, sweetener and vanilla. When it is well mixed, stir in chopped hazelnuts.
2. Form the mixture into balls, press flat with palms and place on dehydrator screens.
3. Dehydrate 1 hour at 145, then reduce to 116 and dehydrate for at least 5 hours or until desired dryness is achieved.

Servings: 24

**Cooking Times**
Total Time: 6 hours

**Nutrition Facts (per serving)**
Carbs: 7g
Fiber: 3g
Protein: 3,5g
Fat: 13g
Calories: 143

# Minty Galettes

**Ingredients**

3 cup coconut butter, melted

1 cup coconut, shredded

3 Tbsp.p coconut oil melted

3/4 tsp. pure peppermint extract

2 Tbsp.p cacao powder

**Directions**

1. In a bowl, mix together, 1 tablespoon of coconut oil and peppermint extract, shredded coconut and melted coconut butter.
2. Pour coconut butter mixture into mini muffin tins by filling half way. Put in refrigerator for about 20 minutes.
3. In a separate bowl mix together 2 tablespoons coconut oil and cacao powder.
4. After 20 minutes remove muffin tin from refrigerator and pour each with cacao mixture.
5. Return to refrigerator for 3-4 hours. Ready!

Servings: 18

**Cooking Times**

Total Time: 20 minutes

**Nutrition Facts (per serving)**

Carbs: 0,5g

Fiber: 0,3g

Protein: 0,25g

Fat: 11g

Calories: 93

# Peppermint Ice Cream Balls

## Ingredients
1 1/4 cup seed butter
1 tsp. peppermint extract
1 1/2 cups coconut oil
1/2 cup sweetener (liquid or granulated)
2 tsp. organic vanilla extract
1/4 tsp. salt

## Directions
1. First, in a small saucepan melt the coconut oil.
2. In a blender add all remaining ingredients and add melted coconut oil. Blend it until smooth well.
3. With the teaspoon grab the coconut mixture and make the 25 coconut balls.
4. Place the balls into a baking sheet and freeze until solid. Keep refrigerated.

Servings: 25

## Cooking Times
Total Time: 10 minutes

## Nutrition Facts (per serving)
Carbs: 8g
Fiber: 1.2g
Protein: 2.25g
Fat: 19g
Calories: 202

# Pistachio Masala Delights

**Ingredients**

1 cup almond butter, melted
1/4 cup ghee
1 cup coconut oil
1/2 cup cocoa butter
1/4 cup pistachio nuts
1 Tbsp. coconut milk
1 Tbsp.p pure vanilla extract
2 tsp. Masala chai (a flavored tea beverage made by brewing black tea with a mixture of aromatic Indian spices and herbs)

**Directions**

1. In a small saucepan melt the cocoa butter over LOW heat.
2. In a large bowl add all ingredients (except the cocoa butter and pistachios).
3. Use a hand mixer and mix well (on HIGH) all ingredients until the mixture combine evenly. Add in the melted butter and continue to blend for 1-2 minutes more.
4. Transfer the mixture to greased and paper lined pan. Sprinkle with chopped pistachios and refrigerate for at least 5 hours.

Servings: 32

Cooking Times
Total Time: 15 minutes

**Nutrition Facts (per serving)**

Carbs: 0,4g
Fiber: 0,1g
Protein:  0, 27
Fat: 17g
Calories: 147

# Raspberry Heaven Squares

**Ingredients**
3 Tbsp. heavy cream
1/4 cup coconut oil, melted
8 oz. cream cheese, softened
1/4 cup coconut oil, melted
3 tsp. raspberry extract
1/2 cup powdered Erythritol
pinch salt
few drops of natural red food coloring

**Directions**
1. Prepare the parchment lined baking sheet.
2. In a bowl, with the hand mixer, blend the cream cheese and sweetener together.
3. Add the raspberry extract, natural food coloring cream, salt and raspberry extract and continue to blend.
4. Add in the coconut oil and continue to blend until it's smooth and creamy.
5. Refrigerate this mixture for 1 hour.
6. When ready, make 48 small balls from batter and place into a prepared parchment lined baking sheet. Place it in a freezer for 2 hours.

Servings: 18

**Cooking Times**
Total Time: 15 minutes

**Nutrition Facts (per serving)**
Carbs: 0,6g
Fiber: 0g
Protein: 0, 77
Fat: 12g
Calories: 101

# Slow Cooker Pecan Nuts

**Ingredients**
2 cups Pecans nuts, halves
4 Tbsp. almond butter
1 cup Stevia or any other natural sweetener
1/4 tsp. ground ginger
1/4 tsp. ground allspice
1 1/2 tsp. ground cinnamon

**Directions**
1.  In a 4-quart Slow Cooker stir the Pecans nuts halves and almond butter until combined.
2.  Add Stevia or any natural sweetener of your choice and stir well.
3.  Transfer to a bowl, combine spices and sprinkle over nuts.
4.  Cover and cook on HIGH for 15 minutes. Turn to LOW and cook uncovered for about 2 hours, or until the nuts are a little crispy.

Servings: 8

**Cooking Times**
Total Time: 2 hours and 15 minutes

**Nutrition Facts (per serving)**
Carbs: 3,6g
Fiber: 2,3g
Protein: 2,9g
Fat: 14g
Calories: 140

# Strawberry Cream-cakes

### Ingredients
5 strawberries
1/2 cup heavy cream
5 Tbsp. butter
5 Tbsp. coconut oil
3 Tbsp. Truvia (or any favorite sweetener)
1 peace dark 100%, sugar free chocolate

### Directions
1. In a bowl, mix heavy cream and the strawberries.
2. With a help of an immersion blender, blend together heavy cream and strawberries.
3. In a separate bowl, add granulated sweetener and the butter; melt butter mixture in the microwave about 30 seconds.
4. Add the butter mixture to a heavy cream and strawberries and blend well.
5. Spoon mixture into your favorite molds. Freeze at least 30 minutes; the longer, the better.
6. Remove mixture from the mold, place on wax paper and melt one piece sugar free chocolate.
7. Pour melted chocolate over the cream and return to freezer for another 30 minutes.

Servings: 12

### Cooking Times
Total Time: 1 hour and 10 minutes

### Nutrition Facts (per serving)
Carbs: 0,6g
Fiber: 0,08g
Protein: 0,3gr
Fat: 16g
Calories: 138

# Strawberry Muffins

**Ingredients**

3/4 cup cream cheese, softened
1/4 cup butter, softened
1/2 cup strawberries, fresh or frozen
1 Tbsp.p pure vanilla extract
10–15 drops liquid Stevia

**Directions**

1. In a mixing bowl, place the butter and the cream cheese and eave at room temperature (about 45min) until softened. Do not microwave the butter!
2. In a separate bowl place the strawberries and mash using a fork.
3. Add the liquid Stevia and vanilla extract and mix well. Add the strawberries to the bowl with softened butter and cream cheese. Whisk until all ingredients are well combined.
4. Pour the strawberry mixture into muffin silicon molds. Place in the freezer for about 3-4 hours.
5. Before serving, unmold the strawberry muffins and place on a serving dish. Keep refrigerated.

Servings: 10

**Cooking Times**

Total Time: 10 minutes

**Nutrition Facts (per serving)**

Carbs: 1,5g
Fiber: 0,2g
Protein: 1,15g
Fat: 11g
Calories: 107

# Walnuts Choco Fat Bombs

**Ingredients**

1/3 cup heavy cream

1/2 cup cocoa butter

1/2 cup pecans, roughly chopped

1/2 cup coconut oil

4 Tbsp. cocoa powder, unsweetened

4 Tbsp. Swerve, Stevia or Erythritol sweetener

**Directions**

1.  In a microwave dish, place cocoa butter and coconut oil together. Use the defrost setting on your microwave and melt in microwave stove for 10-15 seconds.
2.  Add in cocoa powder and whisk well. Pour mixture into a blender with sweetener and cream and blend for 3-4 minutes.
3.  Place silicone molds onto a sheet pan and fill halfway with walnuts.
4.  Pour the mixture with walnuts and place in refrigerator for 6 hours.

Servings: 10

**Cooking Times**

Total Time: 10 minutes

**Nutrition Facts (per serving)**

Carbs: 2,23g

Fiber: 1,25g

Protein: 1g

Fat: 29g

Calories: 150

# Almond Butter Cake with Choco Sauce

### Ingredients
1 cup almond butter or soaked almonds
1/4 cup almond milk, unsweetened
1 cup coconut oil
2 tsp. liquid Stevia sweetener to taste
Topping: Chocolate Sauce
4 Tbsp. cocoa powder, unsweetened
2 Tbsp. almond butter
2 Tbsp. Stevia sweetener

### Directions
1. Melt the coconut oil in room temperature.
2. Add all ingredients in a bowl and blend well until combined.
3. Pour the almond butter mixture into a parchment lined platter.
4. Place in refrigerator for 3 hours.
5. In a bowl, whisk all topping ingredients together. Pour over the almond cake after it's been set. Cut into cubes and serve.

Servings: 12

### Cooking Times
Total Time: 5 minutes

### Nutrition Facts (per serving)
Carbs: 9,8g
Fiber: 2g
Protein: 5,8g
Fat: 23,3g
Calories: 273

# Choco Almond Candy's

### Ingredients
3 Tbsp. cocoa powder, unsweetened
1 cup almond butter
1 cup organic coconut oil
3-4 Tbsp. sweetener to taste
Splash of almond extract (optional)

### Directions
1. In a saucepan over medium heat, melt coconut oil and almond butter. Stir in cocoa powder and sweetener of your choice. Remove from heat and add almond extract.
2. Pour almond mixture into silicone candy molds. Freeze or refrigerate until set.
3. Before using remove from molds and store in a fridge in an air tight container.

**Servings**: 24
Cooking Time: 10 minutes

### Nutrition Facts (per serving)
Carbs: 0,4g
Fiber: 1,22g
Protein: 0,5g
Fat: 9,6g
Calories: 75

# Chocolate-Coconut Layered Cups

### Ingredients
*Bottom Layer:*
1/2 cup coconut butter
1/2 cup coconut oil
1/2 cup unsweetened, shredded coconut
3 Tbsp. powdered sweetener such as Splenda or Truvia

*Top Layer:*
1/2 cup cocoa butter
1 oz unsweetened chocolate
1/4 cup powdered sweetener such as Splenda or Truvia
1/4 cup cocoa powder
1/2 tsp. vanilla extract

### Directions
1. Prepare a mini-muffin pan with 20 mini paper liners.
2. **For the bottom layer:**
3. Combine coconut butter and coconut oil in a small saucepan over low heat. Stir until smooth and melted then add the shredded coconut and powdered sweetener until combined.
4. Divide the mixture among prepared mini muffin cups and freeze until firm, about 30 minutes.
5. **For the top layer:**
6. Combine cocoa butter and unsweetened chocolate together in double boiler or a bowl set over a pan of simmering water. Stir until melted.
7. Stir in the powdered sweetener, then the cocoa powder and mix until smooth.
8. Remove from heat and stir in the vanilla extract.
9. Spoon chocolate topping over chilled coconut candies and let set, about 15 minutes.
10. Enjoy!

Servings: 10

**Nutrition Facts (per serving)**
Carbs: 2,7g
Fiber: 1,5g
Protein: 1g
Fat: 27,5g
Calories: 247

**Author Notes**
Chocolate contains antioxidants known as polyphenols. Polyphenols play an important role in the prevention of degenerative diseases such as cancer and cardiovascular diseases.

# Chocolate-Walnut Squares

**Ingredients**
1/2 cup coconut oil
1 oz cocoa powder
1 Tbs sugar substitute
1 oz walnut pieces
1 Tbs tahini paste
Walnut halves for topping the fat bombs

**Directions**
1. Warm the coconut oil in the microwave until melted.
2. Add the remaining ingredients and stir until well combined.
3. Pour into silicone ice cube trays and refrigerate until almost set.
4. Once almost set, add walnut halves to the top of each fat bomb.
5. Return to fridge until firm.
6. Remove from silicone molds and store in an airtight container in the fridge for up to a week.

**Servings:** 14

**Nutrition Facts (per serving)**
Carbs: 2,5g
Fiber:1g
Protein: 0,7g
Fat: 10g
Calories: 88,5

**Author Notes**
Walnuts have been touted as one of the world's most healthiest foods. Research shows that walnut consumption may support brain health and improve cell function. They contain a good amount of healthy omega-3 fats and are delicious to boot!

# Coconut and Matcha Truffles

### Ingredients
*For the truffles:*
1 cup firm coconut oil (refrigerate if necessary)
1 cup coconut butter
1/2 cup full fat coconut milk, refrigerated overnight
1/2 tsp. matcha green tea powder
1/4 tsp. cinnamon
1/4 tsp. sea salt
1 tsp. pure vanilla extract

*For the truffle coating:*
1 cup finely shredded, unsweetened coconut
1 Tbs matcha green tea powder

### Directions
1. Combine all of the truffle ingredients in a medium sized mixing bowl. Note that it's very important for your coconut oil be firm so send it to the fridge for a little bit if you have to. Same goes for the coconut milk - the thick cream will rise to the top and coconut water will sink to the bottom. While it's not mandatory that you use only the cream part, your milk should be very firm when you use it so make sure that you cool the can overnight.
2. Mix on high speed with a hand mixer, until light and fluffy, then place in the refrigerator to firm up for about an hour.
3. While the truffle mixture is firming up, combine the shredded coconut and matcha powder together in a large, shallow dish. Set aside.
4. With the help of a small cookie scoop form the cold truffle mixture into 32 little balls, roughly the size of a ping pong ball.
5. Roll the balls quickly between the palms of your hands to shape them into perfect little spheres, then drop each ball into the coconut/matcha mixture and roll them until completely coated.
6. Transfer your finished fat bomb balls to an airtight container and keep refrigerated for up to 2 weeks.
7. These can be eaten straight out of the fridge but taste best when you let them sit at room temperature for 10 to 15 minutes before to eat them.

Servings: 32

**Nutrition Facts (per serving)**
Carbs: 0,6g
Fiber: 0,3g
Protein: 0,2g
Fat: 14g
Calories: 123

# Coconut-Raspberry Fat Bombs

**Ingredients**
1/2 cup coconut butter
1/2 cup coconut oil
1/2 cup freeze dried raspberries
1/2 cup unsweetened shredded coconut
1/4 powdered sugar substitute such as Swerve or Truvia

**Directions**
1. Line an 8"x8" pan with parchment paper.
2. In a food processor, coffee grinder, or blender, pulse the dried raspberries into a fine powder.
3. In a saucepan over medium heat, combine the coconut butter, coconut oil, coconut, and sweetener. Stir until melted and well combined.
4. Remove pan from heat and stir in raspberry powder.
5. Pour mixture into pan and refrigerate or freeze for several hours, or overnight.
6. Cut into 12 pieces and serve!

Servings: 12

**Nutrition Facts (per serving)**
Carbs: 3,2g
Fiber: 0,8g
Protein: 0,3g
Fat: 18g
Calories: 169

**Author Notes**
Raspberries contain antioxidants such as Vitamin C, quercetin and gallic acid which help to prevent circulatory disease and age-related decline. They are also high in ellagic acid which has been shown to have anti-inflammatory properties.

# Peanut Butter Fudge

**Ingredients**
1 cup all natural creamy peanut butter
1 cup coconut oil
1/4 cup unsweetened vanilla almond milk
a pinch of coarse sea salt
1 tsp. vanilla extract
2 tsp. liquid stevia (optional)

**Directions**
1. In a microwave safe bowl, soften the peanut butter and coconut oil together. (About 1 minute on med-low heat.)
2. Combine the softened peanut butter and coconut oil with the remaining ingredients into a blender or food processor.
3. Blend until thoroughly combined.
4. Pour into a 9X4" loaf pan that has been lined with parchment paper.
5. Refrigerate until set. About 2 hours.
6. Enjoy!

**Servings:** 12
**Cooking Times**: 15 minutes

**Nutrition Facts (per serving)**
Carbs: 4,25g
Fiber: 1,3g
Protein: 5,4g
Fat: 29g
Calories: 284

**Author Notes**
Coconut oil has a multitude of health benefits including improving glucose tolerance and decreasing risk of cardiovascular disease.

# The High Fat Low Carb Diet Lifestyle Changes

The High Fat Low Carb Diet standards state that the food you eat should elicit a healthy hormonal response in your body.

The hormonal system is like a beautifully constructed web of different hormonal reactions that in turn propel some other actions which are influenced by factors in your food choices, lifestyle choices, and health and stress levels.

The hormonal system chemical courier service in your body. Imagine your hormones needing clear instructions to arrive at their destination. Whatever message they receive is exactly how they react.

Hormones like cortisol, insulin, estrogen, ghrelin. Leptin, testosterone and serotonin among other hormones are all affected by what you eat, your weight, sleeping habits, health history and how you manage stress.

We all want a healthy and normal appetite, stable blood sugar levels, a healthy sex drive, ability to manage stress well and a healthy thyroid. But, let's be real – this is easier said than done.

While you may not be able to control all your hormonal responses, you can at least do your best to take care of your hormonal system.

Here are some simple dietary and lifestyle choices to balance and take care of your hormonal system.

## Take some time out to plan your day

Before you start on your plan, it's important to realize that you don't have to do everything at once or in the same day, scheduling your week over the weekend will allow you to handle your work, customize your High Fat Low Carb Diet meal plan, do a work out and relax, all within 24 hours.

You can also take a few minutes every evening to go through tomorrow's program to ensure that all the meals are in check, your workout, meditation and sleep time are in check and you still have some time to relax.

Look at your plan as a road map that is supposed to guide you on this amazing journey of change. Don't stress too much about it. In fact, look at it like an adventure that is going to impact positively on your life.

Be specific with every plan you make and most of all, be realistic. If your plan is to lose weight; how much weight do you want to lose and within what time period?

Remember, failure to plan is planning to fail!

## Spend less time on the scale and counting calories

The High Fat Low Carb Diet is so much more than losing weight. To focus on how you are faring on the weighing scale and spending every extra minute counting your calories will make you miss out on the lifelong benefits and dramatic health changes that the High Fat Low Carb Diet has to offer.

However, we encourage you to weigh yourself before starting the program and right after the 30 days so you can see the real tangible results of your health efforts and the results of ditching all the inflammatory foods.

## Small but sure

The best way to meet your goals is to start small by setting daily goals then let these transform into weekly goals. For example you can choose to replace your desserts with a healthy High Fat Low Carb Diet snack or dessert for starters.

## Cultivate healthier life habits

If you look at all the amazing things your body can accomplish, there is no question about the fact that your body is a temple. But, so many are the times when you treat like a wood shed instead. How so? Have you ever eaten an entire box of pizza by yourself within minutes?

Well, cultivating healthier habits is the best way to honor your body and to get the maximum benefits of the High Fat Low Carb Diet. In addition to eating fresh, natural and whole foods, get enough sleep – at least 7 hours, go for massages, practice square breathing and other breathing exercises, be one with nature by going outdoors for meditation and relaxation, drink fresh spring waters, take good care of your skin, teeth and bones by going for regular check-ups, etc.

## Drop one bad habit at a time, don't go cold turkey!

We acquire bad habits over the course of time and so does replacing them with healthy habits this is the surest way to success. Take it one habit after another until finally you start leading a pure High Fat way of life.

### Implementing an exciting exercise regime

Exercising doesn't necessarily meaning going for a morning run or hitting the gym for weight exercises. Exercise is what you make it and it should resonate with your greatest passion. Do you love dancing? Sign up for dance fitness classes. Are you more of a spiritual person? Yoga fitness classes will work perfectly for you.

Are you an outdoorsy person? Going for a run in the great outdoors, a hike or rock climbing will suit you perfectly...

If exercise for you feels like a life sentence, then clearly you are doing the wrong exercise. Look deeper within you and determine what you love doing most then go for a fitness routine that's as close to your passion as possible. This way, you will have a blast as you lose all the extra pounds and this will also serve as a great de-stressor.

### Remember...

The better you aim for a balanced lifestyle and food program, manage your stress, take care of your blood sugar levels, the better of your hormones will function. The reason for this is because all of these things propel off of the other, so emphasizing on natural, unprocessed food, getting adequate sleep, finding the perfect exercise regimen for you are some of the most positive and influential things that you have control over and that you can make right for the sake of your health.

### Most importantly...

Your body is a temple that deserves to be well taken care of and nourished. Make your health your priority and you will always make the right choices for your body.

The High Fat Diet is the epitome of how you should feed your body. Don't be too hard on yourself either if you slip. Just pick yourself up and resume from where you left of. With time you will find that you will no longer crave junk and over-processed food.

Your body will be so in tune with the High Fat Diet you will only want to eat what you are sure is providing positive nutrition to your body.

In the High Fat Diet, we have nothing like cheating as all our foods are super tasty and super nutritious. The only thing you need to do is to commit to this diet to allow your taste buds to adjust so you can start craving healthy apple chips instead of the fat laden potato chips in food stores.

# Conclusion

Thank you again for purchasing this book!

I hope this High Fat Low Carb cookbook helps you understand the High Fat Low Carb diet dynamics and principles, why you should do it and how it's going to change your outlook on food and healthy living.

The next step is to get into the right frame of mind and decide that it's time to take charge of your eating habits and your entire life in general.

Even if you have never tried the High Fat Low Carb before, after the 30 days, you will be kicking yourself for having not discovered this sooner.

I hope it was able to inspire you to clean up your diet and ditch the high-carb, low nutrient, toxic food that we, as a society, have come to accept.

The High Fat Low Carb diet is definitely a change in lifestyle that may be difficult at times, but by making these changes, you'll discover increased energy, decreased hunger, and a boosted metabolism.

I encourage you to share these recipes with family and friends, tell them about this book, and let them know that a High Fat Low Carb Diet can be delicious and nutritious.

Finally, if you feel that you have received any value from this book, then I'd like to ask if you would be kind enough to click on the link below and leave a review on Amazon to share your positive experience with other readers.

It'd be greatly appreciated!

51931762R00205

Made in the USA
San Bernardino, CA
06 August 2017